IT'S NOT TRANSPHOBIC TO SAY YOUR DAUGHTER IS A GIRL

The Wise Lesbian Guide For Progressives

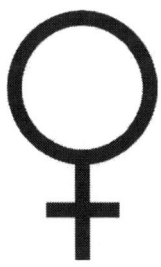

AMBER ALT, PH.D., MSW

It's Not Transphobic To Say Your Daughter Is A Girl

Copyright Amber Alt 2023
Next Generation Books

ISBN: 978-0-9826053-5-6 (Audio Book)
ISBN: 978-0-9826053-6-3 (Paperback)
ISBN: 978-0-9826053-7-0 (ebook)

All rights reserved. No part of this book may be reproduced or transmitted in any form or by any means, electronic or mechanical, including photocopying, recording, or by an information storage and retrieval system - except by a reviewer who may quote brief passages in a review to be printed in a magazine or newspaper - without permission in writing from the publisher.

While the author have used their best efforts in preparing this book, they make no representations or warranties with respect to the accuracy or completeness of the contents of this book. The advice and strategies contained herein may not be suitable for your situation. You should consult with a professional where appropriate. Neither the publisher nor author shall be liable for any loss of profit or any other commercial damages, including but not limited to special, incidental, consequential, or other damages.

CONTENTS

Chapter 1: It's Not You, It's the Ideology 1

Chapter 2: The Old Homophobia in the Emperor's New Hospital Scrubs . 11

Chapter 3: Institutional Capture. 21

Chapter 4: When Gender Affirmation Means Sex Destruction 31

Chapter 5: Brave, Empathic, No-Nonsense, Trustworthy Strategies for Shielding Your Daughter 49

Resources 67

And ain't I a woman? Look at me! Look at my arm! I have ploughed and planted, and gathered into barns, and no man could head me! And ain't I a woman? I could work as much and eat as much as a man - when I could get it - and bear the lash as well! And ain't I a woman? I have borne thirteen children, and seen most all sold off to slavery, and when I cried out with my mother's grief, none but Jesus heard me! And ain't I a woman?

— **Sojourner Truth**

CHAPTER 1

It's Not You, It's the Ideology

Unfortunately, as the world now knows...thousands of vulnerable young people became victims of what was, in effect, a vast medical experiment. It involved powerful drugs with potentially life-changing consequences despite a lack of data to support their use or safety long term, while some clinicians and therapists appeared to be in thrall to increasingly strident trans activist organisations that wielded undue influence over treatment protocols.

— Kathryn Knight, Daily Mail, 16 May, 2023,

When you're used to being on the right side of history—to seeing yourself as someone who's in the business of bending the moral arc of the universe towards justice—it's really hard to suddenly be called a bigot and lumped in with your political enemies.

— Helen Joyce, Joyce Activated newsletter, 31 March, 2023

Welcome. I'm glad you're here.

I wrote *It's Not Transphobic to Say Your Daughter Is Girl: The Wise Lesbian Guide for Progressives* for parents of girls — particularly parents of girls and young women turning toward medical interventions for relief from emotional distress around their bodies, their lives, and what it means to be a woman in the 21st Century. I'm especially hoping to reach politically progressive or liberal parents who themselves suffer emotional pain and conflict around their daughter's cross-sex identification and desire for medical interventions to change appearance. Politically progressive parents face special struggles to make medically safe decisions related to their daughters' welfare that also align with their political, ethical, and moral commitments.

If you are such a parent, you're right to ask questions. I know you are worried, frustrated, demoralized, confused, frightened, and exhausted—especially frightened and exhausted. You also likely feel very alone, particularly if you live in the United States and align yourself with social justice movements and causes. Because of the political dialectic here, progressive adults like you can feel very conflicted about opposing the medicalization of gender non-conforming children. Your progressive friends and family may view the medicalization of children, adolescents and young adults as, well, progressive. When you express reservations, they may accuse you of being manipulated by right-wing Republicans, being a transphobe, or both.

Critical thinking isn't transphobic. It usually also isn't a hallmark of right-wing Republican politics. If you want to safeguard your daughter's physical health and safety, her mental health, her financial security, and her future, you must ask the difficult questions despite enormous pushback. The fact that parents feel unsafe to ask questions, to challenge the currently dominant narrative, and to protect their daughters' bodies from invasive procedures not justified by medical evidence of pathology should signal to progressive parents that you must, indeed, double down.

I hope this small book will reassure you that you must cut through the political spin around this issue, focus on science and material reality, and do what you can to prevent ideologically-driven medicine from destroying your daughter's body. Liberal, radical, and progressive values don't advocate destroying the health of a child, making her a lifelong medical patient, complicating her mental health, or setting her up for disability, immense medical debt, and unnecessarily complicated experiences with sex and relationships.

If you consider yourself a feminist, an ally of lesbian and gay people, an environmentalist, or an advocate for children or for people with disabilities, you must ask serious questions about using the products of big pharma and corporate medicine to solve a problem largely manufactured by these institutions. Any progressive parent should ask whose interests are served as the gender industry transforms healthy young people into patients with shocking levels of medical dependency and disability. We must ask how marketing medically unnecessary hormonal and surgical interventions has made them such a hot commodity.

In this book, I will speak very plainly and directly to you about trans ideology and how you, as an adult, can work to loosen its grip on the girl or young woman you love. I will map out the misogynist and homophobic backstory that paved the way for the pathologizing of kids who don't conform to sex-role stereotypes or conventions, many of whom will grow up to be happy gay and lesbian adults if they are allowed to experience a normal course of development through adolescence. I hope that by providing you with this material, you will feel reassured that the questions you're asking are legitimate. I hope you will feel empowered to resist the tenets of trans ideology that have become pervasive in our institutions. And I hope you will have strategies for keeping your child safer, and knowing where to find other support and resources that will expand on what we begin here.

Before we go forward, you're probably wondering who I am and how I know something about this.

I am both a sociologist and a clinical mental health worker. As a sociologist, my work centers on feminist analyses of LGBT lives and movements, on violence against women and other hate crimes, and on the social construction of mental health diagnoses that stigmatize homosexuality and gender non-conformity, such as Gender Identity Disorder and Gender Dysphoria. My career in sociology has included not only teaching and research, but also applied work in what is now called Diversity, Equity, and Inclusion. I've published work on Gender Identity Disorder, lesbian and bi women's identities, and hate crimes policies, and have taught courses on sex and gender, including a class on LGBTQ mental health. After a long stretch of time in higher education, I decided to expand my skill set and train in mental health.

As a clinician, I have studied personality disorders and suicidality, and treated people suffering from both situations. I've worked in medical settings including in emergency rooms, where I spent several years assessing patients for suicide risk, including gay, lesbian, and trans-identified youth. In my private practice, I've worked with adults in many crazy-making situations in which they have been gaslighted and manipulated — led to believe things that are not true by people who benefit from selling deception. I've trained other clinicians and students in personality disorders, assessing suicide risk, and in working with trans-identified youth — most of whom in previous cohorts have grown up to be gay or lesbian adults. I've supported adults through the transition process and continue to provide therapeutic support to trans adults. Like the incredibly brave and principled Jamie Reed, the author of a 2023 *Free Press* expose essay entitled "*I Thought I Was Saving Trans Kids; Now I'm Blowing the Whistle*," I like to consider myself left of Bernie Sanders. It is because of this history, not in spite of it, that I decided to write this book urging you to do what you can to preserve your daughter's choices. I wish I had written it sooner.

How I Realized the Landslide Was At The Door

Five years ago, I was working in a primary care clinic. That year, 2018, the American Association of Pediatricians instituted guidance that dramatically changed the situation in the United States for kids who don't conform to sex stereotypes, many of whom are likely gay and lesbian youth. Suddenly, and much to the alarm of competent psychotherapists, physicians began to administer experimental puberty suppressing drugs and cross sex-hormones to kids and adolescents who didn't feel comfortable in their bodies, paradoxically setting them on the path to infertility, anorgasmia, osteoporosis, emotional dysregulation, a host of other disabilities and difficulties, and life-long dependency on the medical system.

I observed medical workers present these interventions as a plan of care without advising parents or children that they were experimental, and without advising them that the child or teenaged patient would likely experience a resolution of their dysphoria as they grew through adolescence if they were not medicalized. Given my previous research on the psychiatric medicalization of gay and lesbian people and of gender nonconformity, I found myself startled and deeply alarmed. My first response was incredulity, aware as I was that we — gay and lesbian people, progressive people — have seen this before.

We had known for some time that therapeutic efforts to force kids into gender conformity were ineffective. The impulse behind such efforts often reflected a desire to prevent homosexual adulthoods. The very essence of conversion therapy is this: attempting to make gay and lesbian people heterosexual —- or to appear heterosexual. These efforts have a long track record of failure, and a long record of traumatizing the children and adults subjected to them. Now, medicine was doubling down on gender non-conformity and same-sex attraction in kids by chemically constraining their normal development to make them appear more like the opposite sex — albeit at an incredible price. I witnessed practitioners begin these processes in an amazingly cavalier way, often giving the impression that they were engaged in some sort of merciful, enlightened intervention. Therapists attempting to ask questions were silenced.

As both a sociologist of LGBT experiences and as a clinician, I could barely assimilate what I was seeing. Had something in the science of gender nonconformity changed? When I checked, I discovered stronger evidence than ever from countries that had been medicalizing non-conforming kids — again, most of them gay or lesbian — that medicalization doesn't help and leads to worse medical and mental health outcomes, including higher suicide risk, over the long term. So, nothing had changed in the scientific literature that would justify medicalizing gender non-conforming kids. And yet, I was seeing it and even being asked to participate, to be complicit in causing medical harm to minors suffering no medical illness.

What had changed in the US was not the science but the ideology, fueled by big pharma and corporate medicine, delivered through social media and ideologically captured institutions, including some that historically have been iconic in social justice movements, such as Planned Parenthood, the Human Rights Campaign, and the ACLU. Planned Parenthood, for example, had recently begun to include cross-sex hormones for adolescents and young women as part of its reproductive health model. The Human Rights Campaign, needing a new focus after the legalization of same sex marriage in the United States, saw trans rights as its next focus after appreciating large donations from industries that benefit from trans medicine. It had begun offering medical institutions an HRC seal of approval for adopting so-called gender affirmative care and recognized this as an opportunity to keep the lights on, rather than to declare victory and go on a permanent honeymoon. Social movement scholars know these frame expansion processes and have documented repeatedly how movement organizations pivot when movements achieve their goals, because activist institutions and the people in them have developed vested interests in staying in business that extend beyond their original purpose.

Other writers have further mapped out the financial cooptation of these movement organizations by big money, mostly tied to the pharmaceutical sector and to the biotech industry leaders envisioning a post human/synthetic human/ future. What stunned me, watching physicians confidently starting kids – mostly girls – down the path of medicalization that would cause them irreversible damage, to use the term Abigail Shrier chose for her 2020 book on the topic — was that the physicians justified these practices because they aligned with "The WPATH Standards of Care" or would help the organization "qualify for Human Rights Campaign (HRC) recognition" without apparently ever having pulled back the curtain on what and who WPATH – the World Professional Association for Transgedner Health – and the HRC were, how little interest they had ever had in legitimate research, who sat on their boards, and what these standards reflected. Why were medical institutions allowing such movement organizations to set the course for the administration of experimental interventions, rather than turning to the FDA, the CDC, and the research literature?

I began to recognize the degree of institutional ideological capture that had already occurred, promulgated by these organizations, and that had now trickled down to the local level, coopting institutional practice, medical care, and language. Sociologists know the Thomas Theorem: "that which we take as real is real in its consequences." They who control the terms we use to describe our reality shape our understanding of reality and, consequently, how we navigate the world. In order for physicians to comfortably, even righteously, become complicit in sex-destructive medicine for kids, they had to have experienced a profound shift in reality around sex, gender, and sexuality, fertilized by a transition from scientific to ideological language.

The ideas that kids are "assigned a sex at birth," that they can discover they were mistakenly "assigned the wrong sex," "born in wrong bodies," and must be hormonally and surgically reconstructed on demand in order to reveal "their true selves" had been sold as a natural extension of the gay and lesbian rights movement. Unfortunately, many professionals consuming this narrative don't know that homophobic medicine bolstered by Nazi experimentation had used the very same interventions for decades —- not to liberate, but to persecute gay men and lesbians for our sexuality. They don't know that the idea of sex change as a cure for homosexuality was rooted in the original pseudoscientific formulation of inversion — in the case of women, the idea that lesbians are "men in women's bodies."

As a result, even highly educated people began to believe that "gender" trumped sex; that "pronouns" could not be taken for granted as sex-based; that straight, sex conforming individuals needed to "come out" by "sharing their pronouns;" and that "inclusive care" requires massive changes in language, culture, and practice — no matter how they obscure basic medical knowledge or destroy the safeguards in place to protect the dignity of individuals. That medical practitioners who had cared for thousands of pregnant women and delivered thousands of babies suddenly believed that sex was "assigned" haphazardly at birth represented an incredible and incredibly dangerous ideological capture, because that which we take as real is real in its consequences, even if our belief is fantastical or fanatical.

In the US context, the resulting new medicalization of children found fertile ground in places populated by progressives like me, deeply committed to diversity and inclusivity. Those who started asking questions soon learned to fear cancellation and social ostracization as transphobic, exclusive, or unkind. Others appeared unable or unwilling to think critically about the implications of rushing to medicalize kids uncomfortable in their bodies before they have even had a first crush, explored their distress in psychotherapy, or considered the paradox of how 'being one's true self" could only be realized with expensive and damaging medical interventions. Few have thought to ask whether this was the resurgence of state sanctioned sterilization of gay and lesbian people. Those who have asked have been dismissed or discredited.

Let's Take a breath, Step Back, and Be Brave Together

In a country and culture oriented toward immediate gratification, quick fixes, and avoiding discomfort, we have failed to deeply explore kids' distress and help them resolve it with acceptance, coping, and creativity. Instead of slowing things down, we have accelerated kids toward solutions sold by social influencers and, increasingly, by misguided physicians, therapists, and teachers.

Girls in particular have been vulnerable to the appeal of opting out of womanhood. An explosive increase in girls seeking transition in the US and UK over the last decade tells us that it isn't only young lesbians caught up in the belief that they are literally male, and that looking male as a result of medical intervention will be worth the medical, social, financial, and emotional costs of pursuing it. Previously gender conforming, perhaps heterosexual, girls deeply uncomfortable with the experience of femaleness in a society such as ours are heading onto the trail to trans. Lisa Littman's excellent 2018 research on Rapid Onset Gender Dysphoria (ROGD) in girls helps us to understand social contagion as an additional dynamic in the population of girls — both same sex attracted and not —- seeking transition.

In some ways, the carefully documented and widely observed ROGD girl phenomenon makes the situation more complex. In other ways, it does not add to the complexity at all, because in both groups of girls and young women — those gender non conforming or gender dysphoric since childhood and those with rapid onset desire to transition — are medically healthy. They were all *"born in the right bodies,"* as the title to Dr. Leora Sanger's book reviewing the medical research in this area asserts. They are all caught up in a scandal of medical and social experimentation for which they may pay a lifelong price. Even worse, they are being held accountable for it, because the responsibility for decision making is being transferred to them under the misguided belief that minors have the conceptual capacity and life experience to give informed consent for elective, invasive, experimental procedures.

You, too, as an adult who cares, are caught up in this scandal. You are in a deeply challenging situation. You face the terrifying dilemma of being rejected by your daughter and vilified as transphobic, abusive, and genocidal if you tell the truth OR being complicit in the medicalization of your daughter if you do not tell the truth in an effort to keep the peace and maintain your relationship. Whether you realize it or not now, you and your daughter are similarly stuck: you both are suffering horrible dilemmas created by the tenets of a belief system beyond your control.

You are not alone, though you may have suffered and struggled with this in silence. Across the anglophone world, thousands of moms and dads and growing numbers of doctors and therapists are questioning what's happening and acting to stop it, in children's best interests. Detransitioners, too, are increasingly visible and vocal, and they are asking for accountability from the people complicit in harming them. We all are encouraging the medical system in the US to follow the lead of the other countries that are putting an end to this experimental set of practices.

A late 2022 Washington Post-KFF poll found that 68 percent of American adults oppose access to puberty-blocking medication for transgender children ages 10-14 and 58 percent oppose access to hormonal treatments for transgender kids ages 15 to 17. More than 60 percent said trans-identified males should not be allowed to compete with women and girls in youth, high school, college and professional sports. Nonetheless, two-thirds support bans on transgender discrimination in the military, in K-12 schools, by medical professionals, in getting health insurance, at colleges and universities, at jobs, in the workplace and in housing. These findings confirm that the medicalization of children doesn't signify transphobia or the wish to exclude adult trans-identified people from public life, as much as it reflects a desire for the safeguarding of children against irreversible harm.

As the sociologist C. Wright Mills noted, when one person experiences a troublesome situation, we're looking at a personal problem. When thousands of people experience the same concern, we're facing a social problem. As thousands of girls and their families struggle with medicalization questions driven by trans ideology, we must recognize this as a social problem, one that will not be solved through the unnecessary experimental medicalization of individual bodies. The explosive uptick in girls seeking medical transition tells us we have a social problem. The ignored voices of tens of thousands of self-identified detransitioners tells us that the solution offered by big biotech pharma and corporate medicine is itself a social problem.

In this book, my goals are to tell you the truth, to empower you to become a fierce and protective advocate for the bodily integrity of the child or adolescent you love, and to point you toward an evolving community of therapists, doctors, activists, and writers who will encourage you in making good decisions in support of girls, women, and reality. As a progressive person especially, you need to be able to step out of the Right vs Left dialectic – the binary, as it were — and focus on the empirical, material reality, despite the discomfort that causes. Your daughter is worth the effort.

CHAPTER 2

The Old Homophobia in the Emperor's New Hospital Scrubs

Gender identity theory promotes the idea that a person can be "born in the wrong body," a view adopted by countries such as Pakistan and Iran (where homosexuality is punished by death, but "sex change" is government subsidized as a form of conversion therapy). This attitude may be more common than many realize - whistleblowers from a child "gender" clinic in the UK have stated that "gender-affirming" care is sometimes sought by families who prefer a "transgender" child over a gay child." (citations omitted).

— *WoLF Amicus Brief, Tingley vs Ferguson*

Part 1: The Origins of Nazi Experiments on Homosexuals

In 1919, Magnus Hirschfeld, a wealthy gay physician, sexologist, and human rights campaigner, established in Berlin the Institute for Sexual Science. The Institute, a hybrid clinical, social, and activist space, became an internationally known gathering point for people considered sexual deviants. In particular, the Institute attracted homosexual men, transvestites, and, eventually, transsexuals — many of whom seem to have been, by today's standards, men with autogynephilia.

Hirschfeld sympathized with the period's feminist movement, but focused his medical practice and research on men and male sexuality. The institute housed an activist organization dedicated to repealing the German statute criminalizing homosexuality, Paragraph 195, and became a repository for an extensive mailing list of gay men and others considered deviant that ultimately would come to play a horrifying unanticipated role in the Nazi repression of gay men and lesbians. Hirschfeld worked at both the micro and the macro levels — treating patients and trying to make German society safer for them.

In 1923, Hirschfield introduced the concept of "the transsexual" into the vernacular of the new science of sexology. He used the term broadly — for sex-role nonconformists, for men who felt like women, and for homosexuals. Hirschfeld and other European sexologists also coined another term: "inversion." "Inversion" captured and promoted the idea that people who violate social norms by acknowledging same-sex attraction or resisting sexist prescriptions for behavior are born "in the wrong bodies." In the case of women, this became "men trapped in women's bodies." You'll recognize this pseudoscientific formulation enjoying its renaissance today, to the detriment of children and women a century later, as it underwrites transgenderism in 2023.

With the invention of the concept of transsexual inversion, the Institute began to experiment in the possibility of transforming men into women as a treatment for homosexuality, gender incongruence, and autogynephilia. This line of experimentation hypothesized that some exogenous hormones and surgical remodeling would allow gay men to pass as straight women — and perhaps to become women. The Danish painter Einer Wegener, aka Lili Elbe, became Hirschfeld's most famous experimental subject. Surgeons at the institute first castrated Wegener, then indulged him in three more surgeries — for removal of his penis, the implant of an unknown woman's ovary, and, in a pattern of escalating investment, the implant of an unknown woman's uterus, following the fantasy that it would allow Elbe to become pregnant at the age of 48. Elbe died three months after the final experimental surgery.

One of the surgeons participating in this series of experiments, Erwin Gohrbandt, worked at the time as the director of a women's health clinic, suggesting one possible source of the female reproductive organs implanted in Elbe in the quest to determine if men could be made capable of gestation. Ultimately, he became the chief medical officer of the Luftwafe and the "principle investigator" on perverse Nazi "experiments" at Dachau, no doubt extending the experimentation he had conducted with Elbe on gay men who were identified, rounded up, and interned using the mailing lists Nazis had retrieved from Hirschfeld's clinic. Homosexuality was not only illegal but reviled in Nazi Germany, and its elimination through the murder of same sex attracted men or the pursuit of their theoretical "cure" through hormonal or surgical conversion was sanctioned by the regime.

Gohrbandt was not alone in deeply questionable experimentation on men inclined toward sexual activity with other men, as Elbe had been, as the Nazi eugenics agenda did not align with non-procreative sex or characterological deviance, at least officially. Over the course of the Nazi regime, approximately 100,000 men were arrested for homosexuality and 15 to 50,000 of them were interned in concentration camps. Many of these were subjected not only to extreme forms of abuse, but also to experimentation by so-called Nazi doctors working to "cure" homosexuality or otherwise eradicate it. Many gay men were castrated, as Elbe had been, as part of their treatment for homosexuality, while others were subjected to forced hormone treatments.

Physician and Nazi sympathizer Karl Vaernet had been working to "cure" homosexuality with cross sex hormones in Denmark prior to the war. He ultimately signed a contract with the Nazis that authorized his ongoing experimentation with homosexual men interned at the Buchenwald concentration camp. Surviving records indicate he oversaw the implantation of artificial hormone glands in a number of gay men as part of his experimentation. After the war, Vaernet eventually resettled in Argentina, where he continued this line of research, supported in part by an American chemical manufacturer, until his 1965 death.

"Treating" gay men with cross-sex hormones in an effort to destroy their sex drives and fertility continued in the UK until 1967. Alan Turing, a brilliant mathematician whose code breaking played a pivotal role in ending WWII, and thereby in liberating the Nazi concentration camps where homosexual men, among others, were tortured, was not spared chemical castration when he was convicted of the crime of homosexuality in the UK. [An historical note: when the Nazi camps were liberated, thanks in part to Turing's work, homosexual men were not liberated. Instead, they were transferred to German prisons, to "serve out their sentences" for violating Paragraph 175, the law criminalizing homosexuality.]

The point here should be clear: there exists a long history of trying to eliminate homosexuality through the use of surgical and chemical castration, the use of exogenous hormones, and surgeries designed to reconfigure a person's ability to pass as someone of the opposite sex, often in conjunction with laws that criminalized same-sex sexuality and cross-sex, gender bending behaviors. The deceptively benign sounding "gender affirming care" of the current era is deeply rooted in the 20th Century's homophobia, in eugenics, and in pseudoscientific thinking.

Part 2: Female Inversion: "Men Trapped in Women's Bodies"

> *When she was a teenager, her father caught her reading The Well of Loneliness, the 1928 novel of lesbian love by the English writer Radclyffe Hall. He told her to burn the book. He did so by letter, for he could not bring himself to speak to her.*
>
> — Margalit Fox, on the passing of activist Barbara Gittings

While Hirschfeld focused on homosexuality in Berlin, British sexologist Havelock Ellis paid more attention to the female form of inversion. World War 1 allowed many lesbians to serve in the armed forces and solidify a lesbian culture in which women found each other and empowered themselves to violate the social norm of dependence on men. Same sex desire and same sex romantic, sexual, and social life became more visible, provoking the curiosity of progressives and the outrage of conservatives. Increasingly aware that female partners were not "just romantic friends," sexology began to formulate theories to explain why, given the opportunity, many women would choose other women as their social, sexual, and life partners.

Some sexological theories conceptualized women's same-sex attractions as deviance resulting from 'arrested development." Some explained lesbianism as a sign of "moral degeneration." Havelock Ellis eventually settled on the idea that same-sex attraction reflected natural human variation, but he, like Hirschfeld, couldn't relinquish the idea of inversion, despite the obvious limitations of the idea that lesbianism reflected a "man in a woman's body." The most obvious problem remains with us today: that there is no empirical support for the theory. Beyond this,, the theory focused on women who chose masculine pursuits and female partners, but couldn't explain the homosexuality of women conventional in their femininity. What could possibly explain non-inverted women's attraction to inverts? If two female inverts partnered, were they a gay male couple trapped in two women's bodies? There was no evidence of this, either. Even when other sexologists engaged in rigorous scientific comparisons of the bodies of lesbians with those of heterosexual women, they found no biological, anatomical, or otherwise physiological differences.

Lesbians are not men trapped in women's bodies. Gender non-conforming women are gender non-conforming women. The question of whether inversion explained anything was answered a hundred years ago. In light of this, Ellis concluded that while butch, androgynous, stereotype-defying badass lesbians were shockingly normal females in our embodiment, we had come into the world with a "masculine spirit" a claim that is less verifiable, as it can be neither proven nor disproven, so essentially descends to the level of a religious belief. This is the very same non-scientific, ideologically-based, religious thinking at the center of today's transgender ideology.

Ellis' scientifically untenable theory of masculine spirits tragically trapped in female bodies might have extinguished itself, save for the intervention of British lesbian socialite writer Radcliffe Hall. Hall was quite conservative, a converted Catholic, and taken with spiritualism. She'd had a successful first novel before she turned her attention to her master work, *The Well of Loneliness*, which she envisioned as a story that would evoke sympathy and understanding for the plight of female inverts. Hall liked the heterocentric ideas of the sexologists, with whom she rubbed elbows, felt inspired by the brave lesbian ambulance drivers among her friends, and wanted to see the world be friendlier toward women.

Stephen Gordon, the protagonist of *The Well*, is a strong, tall, smart, woman-loving invert who suffers her share of heartbreak and rejection before she finds love with Mary, who she meets in the ambulance corps. They make friends with another couple, and when one of those women dies, the other commits the obligatory lesbian novel suicide. Stephen worries that "the life" is too much for Mary, and ultimately engages in what is supposed to be understood as an act of butch altruism to manipulate her "normal girl" partner into leaving her for a man – delivering the classic sad lesbian ending. Finally, Stephen, in a phrase anticipating current trans ideology rhetoric, implores God, "Give us also the right to our existence."

Despite its perspective that inversion is god-given, *The Well* isn't an empowering novel. Nor a racy one. We can hear how it presages the idea that lesbians as inverts are doomed to kill ourselves, even though the scientific data don't now and have never supported this, and how it reinforces the pseudo science that lesbians are men stuck in women's bodies.

And yet: the novel, published in 1928, created a furor in England, where the British court declared it obscene because it "defended unnatural practices between women." Diana Souhami, in *The Trials of Radclyffe Hall*, notes that Hall's subversion was that "she dared not to change pronouns to cover up lesbianism, to [instead] write 'she kissed her on the lips.' Where other writers concealed themselves behind allusions.... she spoke out." Souhami reports that the British government determined that the book's use of accurate same-sex pronouns would "blight society's morals and corrupt the young." "At root," she writes, "it was not Radclyffe Hall's book that was on trial, but her prosecutors' ... attitude toward lesbianism."

The novel wouldn't be published again in Britain until 1959. Across the pond, however, *The Well of Loneliness* became a sensation, thanks to its notoriety, and remained the most commonly read novel among lesbians for decades. Although it provided American lesbians a precious touchstone, it also underwrote the ongoing idea that women who defy sex stereotypes are men in women's bodies, and that lesbian life centers on the inevitable loss of our lovers to men, suicides, and social rejection.

Despite persecution, including by institutionalized medicine, during the post-war years, lesbian culture put down roots again. Gay male culture, also ignited by the homosocial experiences of military service, evolved. With greater visibility came greater repression. In the US, laws against same-sex sexuality legitimated harassment of both gay men and lesbians, making us vulnerable to job loss, to family loss, to forced sterilization, institutionalization, and egregious forms of conversion therapy, including hormonal and surgical "interventions."

Remember: Dr. Vaernet, the Nazi physician, was still alive in Argentina and working on ways to eradicate homosexuality, and he was not unique. In 1959, the first edition of the American Psychiatric Association's (APA's) *Diagnostic and Statistical Manual* codified homosexuality as a mental illness, further promoting medical abuses against gay men and lesbians, including chemical castration — similar to the "gender affirming medical care" in the current era — lobotomy, various medically endorsed sexual aversion therapies, and psychotherapy designed to rewire same-sex attractions.

With the emergence of a wave of progressive activism in the late 1960's, gay and lesbian activists recognized the APA's pathologizing of homosexuality as central to our medicalization and oppression. The brilliant lesbian activist Barbara Gittings (whose father told her to burn her copy of *The Well of Loneliness*), in collaboration with gay activist Frank Kameny, designed a multi-layered approach to educating the APA, challenging the APA, protesting the APA, and cleverly trolling the APA with the goal of removing homosexuality as a DSM diagnosis. Half a century ago, in 1972, they staged a powerful intervention at the APA conference in Philadelphia, offering a panel session in which "Dr. Anonymous," a gay psychiatrist, in disguise, made the case for homosexuals. Inside a costume designed by his theater professional boyfriend, the courageous Dr. John Fryer called to account the organization that had quietly looked the other way when gay psychiatrists used the annual meeting to network and offer each other support in a group they jokingly called the GayPA. He pointed out the hypocrisy of the profession and its weaponization against a minority whose natural human variation didn't constitute a mental illness.

That year, the APA removed homosexuality from the DSM.

Part 3: How The New Gender Identity Disorder Displaced the Old Diagnosis of Homosexuality — And Came for The Kids

The APA's decision to eliminate the homosexuality diagnosis, rather than to continue to attempt to eliminate homosexuality itself, represented a revolutionary win for gay men and lesbians. It was a win over the pseudoscience of inversion, the Nazi legacy of experimentation, and efforts to eradicate homosexuality and homosexuals. Barely had it landed, however, when the APA concocted a new diagnosis: Gender Identity Disorder — both of childhood and of adulthood. In the early 1970's, in the midst of the heyday of second wave feminism in the US, the "Free to be You and Me" era, the age of the advent of Title IX and multiple wins for women and girls on multiple fronts, the APA decided that boys who play with Barbie and girls who refuse could, and should, "be treated."

It's clear from the writing at the time that psychologists knew that many gender non-conforming kids would grow up to be gay and lesbian. Now that homosexuality could not be diagnosed and treated per se, the idea behind Gender Identity Disorder of Childhood was to read childhood gender nonconformity as proto-homosexuality and to attempt to prevent homosexual adulthood by treating "sissiness" in boys and "tomboyism" in girls. The original treatment for GID in adulthood was sex-reassignment surgery. The treatment for children was therapy designed to pressure kids into behaviors that aligned with sex stereotypes.

Generally speaking, intensive regressive behavioral therapies didn't prevent gay and lesbian kids from growing up to be gay and lesbian adults, though it did traumatize them. You can imagine that subjecting a gender nonconforming girl to an inpatient psychiatric stay requiring her to put on makeup and a dress every morning and "learn to walk like a girl" as "therapy" for her refusal to enact conventional femininity would do nothing for her self-acceptance, mental health, or appreciation that "femininity" consists of whatever females do.

In the absence of evidence that sex stereotype nonconformity responded positively to the regressive behavioral treatments designed as "gender therapy" by the male psychiatrists practicing it, the Gender Identity Disorder diagnosis persisted. Between DSM IV and V, however, trans activists began to challenge the diagnosis, arguing correctly that gender nonconformity was not a disorder. Unlike Gittings and Kameny and Dr. Anonymous, however, they didn't argue that the diagnosis should be eliminated. Their dream was not to prevent medicine's interference with gender non-conforming people. Their dream was to access sex reassignment technologies without carrying a diagnosis of either a physical or mental illness and without positioning these interventions as elective and cosmetic.

I engaged in participant observation at a trans activist protest of the APA in Chicago in 1997. At a meeting with representatives of the APA's gay and lesbian caucus, I observed the protesters struggling to make the case that trans people were as oppressed as homosexuals had been. Unlike LGB people, however, the trans activists argued against pathologization but for medicalization. They first claimed that gender nonconformity is a "medical condition" like diabetes, and therefore required ongoing access to cross-sex hormones while arguing that unlike diabetes, gender nonconformity shouldn't be seen as an illness. Then they argued that gender nonconformity is like pregnancy — a physical condition that needs medical care —- with the caveat that unlike pregnancy, their medical needs were on-going and life-long. Then they argued that sex-reassignment surgery was comparable to rhinoplasty, which is often elective, while hedging that sex-reassignment is not cosmetic but "necessary" and should proceed from a diagnosable condition — so that US insurers would pay for it.

If anything, the presentation demonstrated transactivists' embrace of the very same medical interventions that had already been used to torture and stigmatzed gay and lesbian people for decades. In DSM 5, the current edition of the psychiatric nosology, GID has been replaced by gender dysphoria, but the same tired sexist stereotypes remain in its criteria, and it's upon this diagnosis that child and adolescent transition now depend. Most kids who are gender questioning or gender dysphoric, or whose caregivers express concern about the child's non-conformity, still see a resolution of their gender concerns in adulthood without medical treatment. Rather than acknowledge this empirical truth, the gender industry has identified a new market in children. Since 2018 in the United States, with the endorsement of the American Association of Pediatrics, physicians in the US have begun to use the same invasive treatments on kids formerly reserved for adults.

The urgency of medicalizing children at younger and younger ages speaks to the awareness that, left to their own developmental processes, most gender questioning kids will begin to feel comfortable in their native sex as they discover sexuality — and deprive the gender industry of customers. There are now more than 100 pediatric gender clinics in the US. Other people have worked out the math of the mind boggling revenue that will be generated by such patients given the life long medical disabilities and dependency many will experience as a result of conditions created by childhood sex destructive interventions.

There never has been any demonstrated biological or anatomical difference between lesbians — female inverts — and heterosexual women, nor between gender non-conforming and conventionally feminine women —- even after a century of looking. There never has been a way to change a member of our sexually dimorphic species into the other sex, despite a century of trying. And despite decades of cutting and shocking, and chemically castrating same-sex attracted people, there has been no effective way of changing sexual orientation or any valid reason for trying. Rather than give up the project, however, psychiatry and medicine have colluded with and been co-opted by big money and clever but truly sinister actors into suspending disbelief, suspending critical thinking, suspending scientific inquiry and allowing themselves to become complicit in recirculating the 20th Century pseudoscientific theory that a girl or woman who defies sexual convention, or who doesn't feel that she is the "right kind of female," must have a male soul that will be liberated by the destruction of her female body.

CHAPTER 3

Institutional Capture

"The party told you to reject the evidence of your eyes and ears. It was their final and most essential command."
George Orwell, 1984.

" A rat in a maze is free to go anywhere, as long as it stays in the maze."
— Margaret Atwood, The Handmaid's Tale.

"This is the oppressors' language, yet I need it to talk to you."
Adreinne Rich, "The Burning of Books Instead of Children."

How did a century old belief system so unmoored from empirical facts and so damaging to women, girls, gay men, and lesbians become so deeply entrenched and institutionalized, making it so difficult and frightening to challenge, resist, or even discuss? How do everyday people stating the known scientific facts that humans are sexually dimorphic, come into the world with an observable sex, and can't change that sex come to feel like Galileo at the Catholic Inquisition for standing firm on the truth that the earth orbits the sun?

How have the progressive, democratic, and feminist ideas that gay people should have the right to exist in society without being castrated or medically maimed, and that kids should be allowed to engage in activities not stereotypical of their sex, been so easily displaced by the practice of "treating" gender nonconformity in kids who likely would otherwise grow up gay? How can it be that some states will investigate parents for refusing their children access to experimental gender medicine and that in other states, parents can lose their children because they do?

How institutional capture occurred in the US and the motivations of the men who have engineered it is beyond the scope of this tiny book. Helen Joyce's book, *Trans: When Ideology Meets Reality*, is an outstanding resource for those interested in the broader issue of institutional capture, as is the *11th Hour Blog* of journalist Jennifer Bilek. Here, I'd like to talk about what institutional capture means for you and your daughter, wherever she may be in her vulnerability to medical transition.

"Institutional capture" refers to the conversion of major institutions to an ideological belief system. Major institutions include the media, government, education, and medicine, with its various specialties, including mental health. When institutions become captured or dominated by trans ideology, they establish practices, policies, and languaging in alignment with the ideology. In doing so, organizations don't only change their way of doing business; they convey to the people who participate in these institutions — students, patients, citizens — that their access depends upon agreeing to, cooperating with, and accepting the terms of the ideology.

We know that ideological capture has taken place when previously normal kinds of conversations become strange, uncomfortable, or nonsensical and asking questions or resisting participation in the ideology risks painful consequences. Those consequences could be job loss, dismissal from care, or the threat of CPS removing your child because you object to her receiving cross-sex hormones. In the case of trans ideology, there have begun to be expectations for compelled speech, silence, or agreement, such as the compelled use of pronouns or the compelled answering of nonsensical questions, such as "what is your gender?" rather than "what is your sex?," even in medical environments, where sex matters.

As I wrote this in the spring of 2023, I happened to hear a National Public Radio news item about the importance of mammograms. It noted that "cis women" and "others assigned female at birth" should receive screenings. The use of "cis" and "assigned at birth" in a national news broadcast about breast cancer indicates that these phrases are meaningful and unproblematic for the journalist using them and conveys an expectation that they are also unproblematic for the listening audience. The adoption of this language by media signals institutional capture and perpetuates and normalizes the cultural diffusion of this language, destabilizing words such as "woman" and "female," and conveying a belief that these categories may be occupied by people of both sexes.

In order for you to free your daughter from trans ideology, you will need to understand the degree of ideological capture in the institutions that are part of your world. The more captured the institution, the more difficult it will be for you to find allies, resources, care, and information that will support your effort to help your daughter reach maturity without trans-motivated medical intervention. The less captured the institution, the less pressure there will be on your child to adopt a trans identity and to engage in sex-destructive elective processes and procedures. If you worry about the degree of capture in the educational and health care systems, the local or state government, the mental health care system where you live, or the media you consume, you will need to evaluate how to loosen their institutional grip on your daughter's self-concept.

Signs of Institutional Capture

Here are some signs that you're dealing with an institution – let's say, a school — with a high degree of institutional capture.

1. Everyone working in the school has a name badge that displays not only a name but also "pronouns," such as "he/him/his" or "ze,zim,zir."

2. The forms you use to enroll your daughter ask for her gender, but not for her sex.

3. The same forms offer options like this in response to the question of gender: "male, female, non-binary, two spirit, other," making sex an identity and subordinate to gender.
4. The school allows "girls with penises," including teachers, to use girls' restrooms and locker rooms.

A note, before we move forward: If you are required to say "girls with penises" in order to determine whether boys and men are allowed in girls' locker rooms, the school is utterly captured. This happens when sex has been accepted as an identity category, which makes it possible for school administrators to say "no boys are allowed in the girls' restroom" because the boys or adult men entering the girls restroom are now officially, by policy and ideology, recognized as girls.

5. Kids are allowed to participate in sports teams congruent with the sex they choose to "identify with" and to use the locker room of that sex.
6. On overnight trips, kids are housed by identity rather than by sex.
7. It becomes clear that teachers discuss their own sex, gender, and sexual identity at school, with students, or ask students to refer to them as a member of the opposite sex.
8. It becomes clear that the school is conveying the beliefs that gender is sex, that sex is assigned, that people of either sex can be the other sex, that girls can have penises and boys vaginas, believing anything else is "hateful" and "transphobic" and saying anything else will result in punishment.
9. The school has penalties for children who "misgender" children or adults by referring to them as a person of the sex into which they were born.
10. The school or teachers in it refer to women and girls as people who menstruate, birth givers, uterus havers, menstruators, etc.

Medical institutions look the same, and medical languaging can look bizarre. For example, I recently reviewed the Medicaid policy manual for a state known as a bit of a trans mecca, and discovered that by policy, "men" are eligible for hysterectomies and "women" are eligible for orchiectomies — the removal of the testicles. A health insurance policy that unselfconsciously authorizes hysterectomies for men is clearly deeply captured, and is one that may make it challenging for you to find doctors who do not code your daughter as a male who needs a hysterectomy to remove the superfluous uterus in her abdomen.

In 2018, heavily funded transactivist groups, including the Human Rights Campaign, successfully lobbied the US government to require any health clinic receiving federal funds to use only electronic health record systems that allow the recording of individuals' so-called gender identity and sexual orientation. In order to keep their contracts with health systems now required to comply with the new directive, electronic health records systems rolled out new Sexual Orientation Gender Identity ("SOGI") menus for use by health care providers. Front line staff and treating medical professionals were strongly encouraged to ask and record each patient's so-called gender and sexual identity.

The resulting initiatives were justified in the name of diversity and inclusivity, even though these identity categories don't convey any relevant medical information about the patient or make physicians any more knowledgeable about how to effectively care for gay and lesbian patients, let alone kids who defy sex stereotypes or are struggling with gender dysphoria. Once a girl is coded as a "trans male" by one provider, this coding follows the patient through all subsequent interactions. That serves both to reinforce the cross-sex social identity of the child, but also creates potential confusion for providers who may begin to see the person as male.

Eventually, you may face a situation in which it is impossible to receive medical care without completing the SOGI section on intake forms, and these forms will require you to treat "gender" as "sex," as many forms in many environments already do. Imagine your daughter being rushed to an emergency room, unable to speak for herself, and being evaluated and treated as male, rather than female. Imagine your daughter literally believing she has become male, as a surprising number of transitioned young people do, and believing therefore that she cannot experience any of the health issues typically of concern to girls and young women. The use of SOGI to code patients as the opposite sex reflects institutional capture, and the top down process is typical of many elements of how trans ideology has been adopted and implemented in the US.

In parallel with this, many state and local governments have adopted or extended conversion therapy bans. This sounds positive at first encounter. Most progressive people are supportive of banning conversion therapy, which historically has been understood as the unethical practice of interventions designed to change a person's sexual identity or orientation —- including chemical castration with drugs like lupron. The Nazi practice of castrating homosexuals, administering exogenous hormones to sterilize them or eliminate sexual desire, or the aversion therapies and lobotomies and egregious forms of psychotherapy to which lesbians have been subjected, fall squarely under the umbrella of conversion therapy — not therapeutic at all.

The new conversion therapy bans, however, prevent or deter therapists and doctors from doing anything other than affirming a cross- sex identity in people who seek counseling about not feeling comfortable in their natal sex. Rather than help a person feel at home in their body, the therapist is directed to assume that the discomfort requires cross-sex medicalization. Through this linguistic sleight of hand, "conversion therapy" in trans ideology means helping the person become comfortable in their body as it is, exploring the roots of their dysphoria and discomfort, and asking the hard questions psychotherapists are trained to ask.

These new conversion therapy bans have had a chilling effect on the practice of psychotherapy with people struggling with questions of sex and sexuality. They have been interpreted by many medical and mental health practitioners as making it illegal to do anything other than immediately and consistently affirm a cross-sex identity in a gender-questioning kid and direct that child toward medical interventions. Note that doing this is, fundamentally, in many cases, gay conversion therapy, given how many gender questioning kids are gay. As far as I know, nobody has yet legally tested whether therapists pushing kids toward medicalization are violating the conversion therapy ban as it was originally conceived – to protect gay and lesbian people.

So — between a health care system that wants to record your daughter as a trans male and then continue to move her along the path to transition, and physicians and therapists who buy into the empirically unsupported ideology or are reluctant to treat her in gender exploratory ways if they are working inside of ideologically captured systems, the path forward will be difficult to navigate. The professionals in places parents might have turned for support, guidance, help and care a decade ago now either have been ideologically captured or are afraid to act in accordance with science and good sense — unless you make it very clear to them you want them to do so.

With trans ideology, institutional capture has occurred slowly, quietly, and in processes that are opaque to most of us. Unlike grassroots social justice movements, policies have been presented by extremely well-funded organizations to governments that have adopted them quietly and begun to enact them largely unopposed – because the general public has been unaware of the changes institutionalized by these new policies.

This is why people feel so shocked and surprised to realize that men convicted of the sexual assault of women are now housed in women's prisons, males are on women's and girls' sports teams, in womens and girls' bathrooms, and have the legal right to proclaim themselves female — because the laws, policies, and deals destroying women's protections in single sex spaces have been made in a top-down manner. The media has largely fallen in line, for example, referring to males who identify as women as female or as women, giving you the impression that a woman killed her neighbors, or her father, or assaulted women at a women's rights speak-out, when the material reality involved males claiming to be women. The policies shaping all of these practices have rolled down, rather than up, as from the social justice movements with which most of us are familiar.

How to Advocate for Your Daughter's Freedom

We will discuss strategies for you to use directly with your daughter in another chapter, but here, I'll offer these recommendations:

Understanding the concept of ideological institutional capture is key for your own clarity. Recognize that not only are you up against the distorted thinking, erroneous beliefs, and reactivity of your daughter; you are also up against ideologically captured institutions that reinforce her distorted beliefs. Had your daughter become indoctrinated by a UFO cult, you would still have an uphill battle in deprogramming and reclaiming her, but you would not usually have to worry that her doctor, teacher, therapist and best friend's mom were going to reinforce her UFO cult belief system or whisk her off to the cult headquarters. Here, with what many parents view as a trans cult or religious ideology, you will need to focus on your daughter and on her exposure to ideology in the institutions with which she has contact. If the process is turbulent, imperfect, and conflict-ridden, try not to give in to despair. Give yourself grace. There isn't a clear handbook for extracting trans ideology from your daughter's thinking or extracting her from medicalization. It's hero's work, and heroes often stumble.

You need to become familiar with the laws in your state related to childhood medicalization, which will be called gender or transgender care or gender affirmative care — the language itself is a sign of ideological capture. You also need to know state and local law and school policy related to educational environments as they relate to trans ideology, gender identity, single sex spaces, pronoun use, and transitioning kids without informing their parents — both via social transition and providing access to medicalizing gender services.

If you are fortunate enough to live in a state that has put the brakes on medicalizing gay and lesbian youth and gender questioning girls, you can breathe a little easier, but not entirely relax. A number of states are establishing themselves as sanctuary states for trans youth, meaning that your minor child could run away to these states and begin the process of medical transition there without your permission or even your awareness — another signal of both institutional capture and the motivations of the industries that expect to make more money than they will lose through the initial medicalization process. The Movement Advancement Project (MAP) maintains a color coded map of "LGBTQ Equality" by state that can be useful in assessing a state's general climate, but doesn't make fine distinctions between laws that protect trans identified people from workplace discrimination and laws that prevent therapists from practicing gender exploratory therapy.

Become brave about asking direct questions to teachers, doctors, administrators, program leaders, and others. For example, you need to ask physicians and therapists questions such as "When it comes to caring for girls who say they are boys, are you required by state or local law, or by your employer, or by a professional organization to affirm a cross sex identity?" "How do you approach caring for kids with trans identities?" Ask schools how many "trans youth" are in the school and how many "trans teachers" work there. The answers to the questions will give you some idea of how captured the institution is.

You can also ask these questions of organizations themselves, writing to the clinical director of a healthcare organization or to the owner of a mental health practice. You might ask "What is your approach to caring for kids who struggle with gender identity?" or "Are you comfortable with gender exploratory therapy as an approach to working with my daughter?" "How much experience do you have working with gay and lesbian teenagers and adults?" How much do you know about the comorbid conditions that can be mistaken as signs of "trans" identities in kids?

There are many responses to institutional capture — avoiding or leaving these institutions, directly challenging these institutions, working to expose the ideological capture, changing these institutions from within, and creating alternative institutions that are not anchored in regressive ideologies. For our purpose here — saving your daughter from trans ideology — the most important focus is on her and shielding her from a pseudoscientific ideology that can drive her toward medicalization, or extricating her from this way of thinking if she's already drawn into it. You don't have to change these institutions right now. Saving your daughter is more than enough.

CHAPTER 4

When Gender Affirmation Means Sex Destruction

"I woke up and realized I'd made the worst mistake of my life."
— **Survivor of elective bottom surgery**

"That's what I hear: 'I have ruined my life. I had a perfectly good body and now it's ruined.'"
— **Lisa Marchiano, therapist to detransitioners, Interviewed in the documentary film No Way Back: The Reality of Gender Affirming Care**

"These vulnerable people were treated incredibly badly by the professionals."
–**Stella O'Mally, founder of Genspect Interviewed in the documentary film Affirmation Generation**

If you read the earlier chapters of this book, you learned about the history of medicine using hormones and surgery to attempt to "cure" homosexuality or effectively eliminate gay and lesbian people ourselves. You learned a bit about the deep historical connections between these approaches and the Nazi regime, pharmaceutical companies, and other nations administering hormones and surgery as either punishment for or cure for same sex desire. And you began to consider the current institutional capture that has re-branded these practices and presented them as therapies that are appropriate, benevolent, medically necessary, and life saving. You've learned that the justification for these practices is based on the pseudoscientific idea that we can be born in the wrong bodies, that this explains same-sex attraction, and that this is a pathology in need of cure.

Between the disturbing backstory and the institutional capture that makes it incredibly unlikely that your daughter won't be exposed to this ideology, I hope it's becoming clear why you personally must step up to protect your daughter's welfare — physical, emotional, social, sexual, and financial—--- from the impact of trans ideology.

Let's review the distortions baked into the ideas about transition, then turn our attention to what is known about the medical risks of sex- destructive interventions, particularly for young people. Because of institutional ideological capture, much of this may be news to you or involve ways of thinking about medicalization that require a shift in your perspective and understanding. Fortunately, though these shifts may be alarming, they will nonetheless likely not require much in the way of mental gymnastics, unlike the Orwellian trans ideology to which we all have been recently exposed.

At the outset, I'd like to assure you that you are absolutely right to be asking questions about whether medical modifications to your daughter's body will improve her mental health, her physical health, her financial future, and her social and romantic life. You are also absolutely right to be skeptical about the idea that modern medicine can make your daughter male. Asking these questions, and having these reservations doesn't make you transphobic. If you haven't asked them previously, you're also not a bad parent. Please be kind to yourself and keep breathing as we enter this difficult territory.

Pulling Back the The Gaslight Curtain

First, I'll remind you that the vast and overwhelming majority of girls uncomfortable with being female experience a resolution of their discomfort around sex, sexuality, and their self-concept by early adulthood, if they are allowed to mature without medicalization. To say it differently: despite the deep discomfort with femaleness experienced by some girls, teenagers, and women, most of us eventually become comfortable in our female bodies and in our womanhood, however we express ourselves or choose to live. This happens even for those of us who spend our childhoods identified as boys and eschewing femininity.

If you do not treat your child's emotional distress over the idea that she is female with social transition, puberty blockers, cross sex hormones, double mastectomy, hysterectomy, or genital surgeries, the odds are great that she will grow up to be a woman eventually comfortable in her own skin. Researchers, therapists, and adults who experienced gender-expansive or gender dysphoric childhoods have known this for decades.

Second, despite the terrifying ideological rhetorical claim that kids who don't conform to sex role conventions and stereotypes will kill themselves if they aren't allowed access to medical interventions, the social science data on this offer it no support. In fact, among kids enrolled in the gender identity disorder service at the UK's now-infamous Tavistock clinic, the rates of suicide among child and adolescent patients who had not received any experimental medical treatment were lower than kids in the general population. Longer term data among the patients still being followed by clinicians practicing the Dutch Protocol, which includes hormones in late adolescence followed by surgery before 20, documents that rates of suicide in this patient population are significantly higher than in the general population, which no doubt includes individuals who experienced gender dysphoria in childhood. Often these tragic losses occur a decade after transition.

If your daughter struggles with suicidality, she needs mental health treatment. (A special note to progressive parents: the idea that mental illness or even mental distress in women should be treated with medical interventions on our wombs, ovaries, or genitals is centuries old, unscientific, and a deeply misogynist expression of victim blame.) While testosterone does often level out a girl's adolescent mood swings for a while, there are other medications and therapeutic practices that also do this, without the negative risks of testosterone. If your child is suicidal, she needs mental health help, first and foremost.

Some detransitioners report that they sought transition because they feared they would kill themselves without it. They worried about this not because they were actually suicidal, but because they believed influencers' deployment of the outdated stereotype of the inevitable lesbian suicide – a la *The Well of Loneliness* — and wanted to avoid it through medicalization —- which, ironically, increases their risk of suicide.

Third, the medical interventions offered as "treatment" for gender dysphoria are experimental. Period. In the US, the drug Lupron is the most commonly used gonadotropin releasing hormone agonist. Lupron is a powerful medication authorized for use in treating precocious puberty in girls, prostate cancer in men, and endometriosis in women. It has also been used to chemically castrate rapists. It is not authorized by the FDA for use as a mental health medication or to treat gender dysphoria.

When it is used to stop sexual development in very young girls prematurely advancing into puberty, physicians use it cautiously and briefly, knowing that the medication often has some very serious negative consequences. When medical professionals use it to stall puberty in kids who are developing normally, they are using this powerful drug experimentally — a fact now acknowledged in several other countries. While off-label use of powerful drugs isn't unheard of, it often happens in the context of clinical trials or valiant efforts to save the life of someone suffering from end-stage illness. Here, physicians are using puberty blockers experimentally to respond to a situation that is not a medical emergency — or even a medical pathology.

The same is true of double mastectomies on healthy breasts, elective hysterectomies, genital surgeries that destroy the architecture and functionality of the vagina and clitoris, involve gruesome skin grafts, urethral resectioning, and in many cases result in life threatening complications. All of this is experimental. All of it involves unnecessary risk. All of it is a misallocation of medical resources and a violation of the hippocratic oath to do no harm. All of it is extraordinarily expensive and sets your daughter up for a lifetime of both medical dependence and medical expense, deeper psychological challenges, various kinds of disability, and a high risk of infertility, sexual dysfunction, and relationship challenges — and yes, an elevated suicide risk.

Fourth, there are no clinical empirical standards for determining that a child is "transgender" — because this identity is not rooted in empirical reality or evidence-based medical assessment. The child's announcement or the parents' endorsement of this identity supersedes the lack of evidence that can be seen on a scan or measured by blood work. When physicians prescribe puberty blockers for premature puberty — an actual medical condition — a child's hormonal profile and physical body indicate that she is entering puberty at 7 or 8. When a child of 7 or 8 or 17 or 18 claims that she is not female, the only evidence is the claim or the report of a feeling. The vast majority of girls reporting the feeling that they are not girls show no physical evidence on exam of being anything other than female; their hormonal profiles are usually typical of females their age. The physician who writes a prescription, is treating an unsubstantiated belief or a set of feelings with a drug not authorized for this purpose.

Consider anorexia as an analogy. Remember that girls struggling with anorexia will often report to physicians that they are overweight or obese, but physicians look at the evidence to assess whether the claim is empirically true, and are able to discern that it is not. The fact that an anorectic girl feels obese doesn't lead a physician to treat her for obesity by helping her lose more weight. Indeed, to do so would be a most unethical form of malpractice. As detransitioners begin to sue medical systems and providers, it becomes clear that prescribers and therapists, in the throes of ideological capture, have underestimated their vulnerability to allegations of unethical conduct in the case of trans medicine, as well.

Fifth: If your daughter is same-sex attracted but fancies herself male and makes irreversible changes to her body so that she can "pass as" male, she will face many challenges in finding a mate. Heterosexual women generally look to date males. Some may stretch their criteria, but many cannot and will not date transmen. Lesbians date women, and some especially fancy "butch" or soft butch women, but not men and not women who hate their female bodies or wish to be seen as male. She may discover that she is not attracted to males who "identify as" women If your daughter is opposite-sex attracted and reconfigures herself as male, she will likely be excluded from the pool of potential male partners attracted to women, but also will find it difficult to partner with gay men — who are same-sex attracted and recognize that your daughter isn't male.

There are certainly transitioned adults who create viable partnerships. Too infrequently, however, are considerations of a girls' relational desires openly discussed and considered as part of conversations about medical transition — unless she is being pressured by a love interest to transition, a dynamic that happens more frequently than you might imagine, due to homophobia. A girl's sexual future needs to be part of the conversation about gender, because the truth is that gender affirmative care destroys or damages sex, and damages sexual functioning, reproductive capacity, and relationship options.

Finally, let's consider for a moment the term "gender affirming care." It has a positive connotation, sounds benign, and is medically vacuous and nonspecific. In trans ideology, everyone is born with a gender that is more significant than biological sex. Theoretically, everyone, therefore, should have access to this "gender affirming care." What would that look like for a boy frustrated that his muscle mass isn't what he would like at 14? Why is such a boy generally not offered testosterone? When women enter menopause and begin to notice physical signs of the hormonal shifts associated with the change, it is not standard to offer us hormone replacement therapy in the US because of concerns about its negative effects, even though HRT, unlike cross sex hormone regimens, replaces what had been typical of this particular women's body. Likewise, girls who notice some unwelcome hair growth at puberty aren't typically offered hormones or even life-saving gender affirming laser hair removal. Nor is this true at menopause. It's not considered medically necessary for mid-life women to receive facelifts or breast lifts or posterior implants or liposuction as part of medically necessary "gender affirming care," no matter how deep the distress over our plummeting body parts may be.

My point: the idea of gender affirming care narrowly focuses on interventions that arguably deepen discomfort with one's natal sex, rather than reduce that discomfort by providing education, relevant clinical testing, and appropriate reassurance about the many ways of being female, the process of puberty and maturation, and psychotherapy for the many difficult experiences that channel girls toward the feeling that they aren't good enough girls or female at all. " Gender affirming care" as a term covers sex destructive medical practices, and reflects a marketing strategy to normalize and even commodify the interventions that it covers.

To summarize these six points: medical science can't provide any evidence of a biological or medical problem that results in "feeling like the opposite sex" and that justifies medical intervention. If you ask a doctor to provide empirical evidence that your child is "trans," they will not be able to provide it. Kids who aren't subjected to sex destructive biomedical treatments are not at higher risk of suicide than the general population, while people who are medically transitioned are, at the ten year mark, far more likely to end their own lives. People struggling with suicidal thoughts and impulses need mental health support, not genital surgery. Most kids who have "cross-sex feelings" turn out to be gay, though some are bisexual or heterosexual, and most experience a resolution of cross-sex identification and gender dysphoria as they pass through puberty and enter early adulthood.

Kids who are transitioned before they have sorted out their patterns of affection and attraction pay a price when it comes to mate selection. "Gender Affirmative Care" is empty, gaslighting, non-medical language that normalizes the idea of gender as a medical concept. The push to treat kids who violate sex role stereotypes, at increasingly younger ages, with increasingly intrusive and damaging approaches, reinforces sex role conventions, stigmatizes and masks homosexuality, and dates back to the debunked century-old old pseudoscientific concepts of inversion — the situation of men trapped in female bodies. Here, in the 21st Century, according to trans ideology, gender non-conforming girls must free the men they were meant to be through the destruction of outward markers of femaleness and internal organs of generation.

Lifting The Gown

In this section, we'll look a little more closely at the medical realities beneath the obfuscating language of the medical procedures that constitute "gender affirming care." For a much more comprehensive review of the medical literature on this topic, read *Dr. Isadore Sanger's Born in the Right Body*.

Humans Don't Come With A Pause Button

Parents make different strategic decisions about social transition, depending on a child's age and the family dynamics, but the picture that has emerged is that social transition increases the likelihood of a child being prescribed puberty blockers, and a course of puberty blockers nearly always results in progression to cross-sex hormones. There is a puberty blocker sales pitch that involves physicians saying that their use, which stops the progression of puberty, buys children and families "time to think" by "hitting a pause button." The impression physicians seem to attempt to give is that puberty blockers are benign and cause no irreversible damage. Patients and parents are led to believe that once the blockers are discontinued, puberty will resume and run its natural course, just on a delayed timeline.

The sociologist Michael Biggs traces the origin of this framing to the Dutch pediatric gender service, which sought to mitigate the idea that children weren't in a position to give informed consent for this treatment. Rather than address the ethical issues involved, the Dutch began to frame puberty blockers as so benign that there was no issue with informed consent from minors. Unfortunately, this is not the case. Puberty blockers are not FDA-approved for stopping puberty in healthy kids, because they risk any number of negative outcomes, including suppressed height for girls, osteoporosis and joint problems, imbalanced brain development, and impaired cognitive development — none of which appear to be reversible. I would note that the idea of "a pause button" is a mechanical analogy and therefore an inappropriate one for an organic, living, breathing, complex organism, such as a developing human girl. She does not have a pause button. This metaphor makes the concept more palatable than comparing blocking puberty to stunting the development of other organisms or putting Spring on hold. It also begins to pathologize puberty. There's a reason for this. Most gender dysphoria resolves in the wake of natural puberty. By preventing patients from advancing through their natural puberty and rerouting them onto a cross-sex path following the use of puberty blockers, their medical momentum toward surgeries and myriad medical challenges accelerates.

Dr. Marci Bowers, the trans-identified physician and public face of WPATH, said on a recent webinar that "100 percent of kids started on blockers" can't experience orgasm. If this is true, rather than a pause in natural development, the impact of blockers is an end to the patient's potential for natural sexual pleasure, along with its other detrimental effects.

The Anabolic-Androgenic Steroid of Body Builders, Russian Athletes, and Gender Affirmative Care for Girls

The perceived benefits of testosterone enjoyed by masculinizing girls include an initial leveling of moods, an increased ability to build muscle, and the redistribution of fat. Many women on "T" experience the chemical interruption of their periods. Their voices drop into a deeper register, which is often irreversible.

The negative impact of testosterone use can include: vaginal atrophy, vaginal tearing leading to discomfort while engaged in every day activities and especially during sex, chronic bacterial vaginosis, chronic or recurrent UTIs, the need for supplemental topical estrogen normally used by menopausal women, male pattern baldness, male pattern weight gain, cardiac issues, and an elevated risk of earlier dementia or Alzheimers, congruent with earlier menopause. Frequently, women following this course will experience pelvic pain that leads to recommendations of hysterectomy. Many suffer chronic urinary incontinence. Some experience clitorial growth that results in friction and pain without apparent sexual benefit. Between blockers and cross-sex hormones, many become sterile.

"Top Surgery" is Double Mastectomy by a Gender Neutral Name

Double mastectomy is also known as "top surgery." Despite frequent claims that women under 18 aren't subject to double mastectomy in the name of trans medicine, a recent report by Komodo Heath initiated by Reuters News revealed that 776 girls between the ages of 13 and 17 with a prior diagnosis of gender dysphoria underwent double mastectomies between 2019 and 2021 in the US — during the height of the coronavirus pandemic. The researchers note that this number is likely an under count, as it includes only those procedures paid for by insurance or taxpayer-funded state medicaid programs.

Survivors of these elective mastectomies report that their negative experiences after mastectomy include pain, temporary disability and dependency, post-surgical complications, loss of sensation across the upper body. the inability to breastfeed, painful scar tissue and unexpected emotional distress — both about the loss of the breasts and about the disfigured appearance that often results. Jamie Reed, a Washington University pediatric gender clinic former staffer, recounted in her stunning *Free Press* expose the day she took a heartbreaking call from a distraught teenager who, a few months after mastectomy, wanted her breasts back.

Hysterectomy: The Surgery Named After Hysteria, Women's Ungovernable Emotional Excess

Hysterectomies predictably result in early menopause, requiring additional hormonal interventions and therapies in women decades before they would have reached natural menopause. Hysterectomy obviously results in infertility and sexual complications, along with an elevated risk of Alzheimer's disease and shortened life span.

"Bottom Surgeries:" Why Some Trans Activists Oppose Legislation Against Female Genital Mutilation

For women, "bottom surgery" is a sanitizing term for two procedures, metoidioplasty and phalloplasty. In metoidioplasty, casually referred to as "mets," a testosterone enlarged clieris is surgically repositioned to create a phallic structure that may range from 1 to 3 inches in length. The patient's labia are surgically altered to create a scrotum. Additional procedures may include grafting tissue from other parts of the body, rerouting and extending the patient's urethra in an effort to integrate it with the neopenis.

Phalloplasty is a more complicated surgery involving a skin graft, usually from the patient's forearm, which suffers a resultant loss of sensation. Surgeons take additional tissue from arms, legs, and sometimes inner cheeks in an effort to construct a tube of skin through which an elongated urethra can be routed. Success rates in terms of sexual and urinary functioning vary. Surgical complications that require ongoing revisions, and ongoing treatment for ongoing infections, are common. Scott Newgent, a former business executive turned activist, has publicly detailed her horrifying, harrowing, disabling experience with medicalization in multiple testimonies in states considering child transition, in a groundbreaking interview in the film "*What Is A Woman?*" and on her website at TREVoices.com.

Survivors of both metoidioplasty and phalloplasty often suffer urinary complications, living long periods of time with suprapubic catheters and dealing with ongoing urinary infections. Other infections related to the complexity and locations of these surgeries often require emergency interventions, revisions, and long courses of antibiotics — at a time in life when a young woman could otherwise be enjoying the pleasures of late adolescence or early adulthood.

It's important to remember medical professionals impose these interventions on bodies healthy at the start. The breasts and wombs and clitori and urethras and forearms and labia are perfectly functional and not in need of medical intervention. Medicine and trans activists frame the exogenous blockers, the exogenous hormones, the surgeries as "medical" and as "care" in their dissemination of the ideology. In 1933 at Hirschfeld's clinic, or in the German concentration camps, or in the clinics endeavoring to "cure homosexuality" while it was still both a crime and a degenerate mental illness, every one of these experimental procedures would have been framed as an effort to eradicate homosexuality or to eliminate gay people through conversion. From the perspective of the people upon whom it was imposed, it was often framed as torture, or as an "option" to which one must submit in order to live beyond an institution. There's a truism in social psychology that the more we invest in something, the more we value it —or at least continue to invest This is well known by fraternities and other organizations and investments with high upfront costs, and by business people who understand the sunk costs fallacy — the tendency to keep investing even when things aren't going well. Between clinical momentum, social pressures, anticipatory socialization, and sunk costs, it can be very difficult for someone who has started down the trail to transition to stop the process. It's important that we make stopping an option and help girls and women who have been medicalized understand they still have choices and are still female.

Many detransitioners report incredible losses when they recognize that transition was an inappropriate choice, or that they were misinformed and ill-advised, inappropriately assessed, or pushed into transition before they had the cognitive capacity and life experience to truly give consent. When they turn to their gender therapists or the gender clinics that supplied them with blockers or hormones or surgery, they are told to look for care elsewhere because they are no longer "transitioning" patients. The trans community, similarly, is reported to harass and degrade detransitioners, seeing them as traitors and betrayers.

When children are started on this series of steps, and accelerated through them, no plan is made for regret or desistance. When gender dysphoric kids are not medicalized, their dysphoria usually resolves post- puberty. If it doesn't, they have a fully developed and still fully functional body about which they have greater maturity to make adult choices, given enough appropriate information, using more mature brains.

Remember — the young people advised to pursue these medical interventions are not intersexed. They are generally medically healthy children, adolescents, and young adults. So, in delivering so-called "gender affirming care," medicine isn't addressing a medical illness.

If Transition Doesn't Solve A Medical Problem, Does It Cure Mental Illness?

If "gender affirmative care" doesn't cure a problem with the body, maybe it cures a problem with the mind, as implausible as this possibility sounds. Girls suffering from anorexia often misperceive themselves to be obese or overweight and are very uncomfortable in their bodies as a result, and girls suffering dysphoria are very uncomfortable in their bodies — much like most girls experiencing puberty are, one way or another. The perception that one is "in the wrong body" doesn't confirm the wrongness of the body, however, anymore than an underweight girl's perception that she is fat confirms that her body is obese. But how does medicalization fare as a mental health intervention?

There is no long term evidence that children or young adults subjected to these interventions are physically or emotionally healthier as a result. A recent large study comparing kids labeled as trans and their siblings confirmed that medical interventions did not improve the mental health of the kids subjected to them. At the end of the study, the trans-assigned kids had increased their use of mental health meds, including powerful anti-psychotic agents, and their suicidal ideation had increased. The findings of this study confirm the findings of other longer-term higher quality data sets, as well as observations from a growing chorus of physicians, psychologists, and detransitioners sounding the alarm in the US, with the hope that we will follow the leads of countries that have systematically studied this issue more closely and discontinued these practices. Post-transition, the completed suicide rate in this population is 19 times greater than that of matched controls who did not transition.

What Happened to "Do No Harm?"

If the risks of medicalizing girls are so high and the poor outcomes so numerous, why haven't you heard more about this from your daughter's physicians or therapists? Why have you felt that your daughter and you have been pushed into, rather than away from, medical interventions as a response to her distress and discomfort? Why must it fall to you to become an expert on a range of subject areas you previously would have turned to professionals for reliable guidance on?

It's important to think systemically here, and to recognize what's happening upstream of where your daughter is today. Upstream is an industry that stands to make a massive profit from her continued travel through the process of medicalization. Medicalization will make her a customer for life, and that will continue to enrich the industry upstream. Similar to the heavy burden of student loan debt and the predatory practices that have saddled many Americans with it for life, the sexual medicalization of children and young adults will obligate them to immense medical debt as they depend on hormones and secondary treatments for the complications of their sexual medicalization.

Before we explore some of the reasons that your daughter's doctors, therapists, and teachers may be encouraging her to slide down the muddy bank or jump into the river, it's important to recognize that as with the opioid scandal, the pharmaceutical industry and corporate medicine benefit from the buy-in of these experts. In order for pediatric gender medicine clinics to be profitable, these industries needed to have confidence that they would have customers, and those customers would be referred by these professionals.

So, why would otherwise trustworthy professionals be putting your child on a path toward devastation, and even shaming you for asking questions?

Many have not thought critically about the information they've been given. In large organizations, professionals rely on institutional authority for guidance on policy and practice and sometimes become complacent. If an organization provides an update that says "the new best practice is to start gender-questioning kids on puberty blockers at Tanner 2, so screen all kids for this" an overworked medical professional may say "got it" and go on about their hectic day. Despite the robust history of egregious medical experimentation and scandal in this country — think here everything from Marion Sims to Tuskegee to opioids —- most medical professionals still trust the institutions in which they have been trained for information.

Most medical professionals also have had minimal education about gay and lesbian history. They particularly know little about the history of medicalizing gay and lesbian people and next to nothing about lesbians and lesbian health and development in particular. Because of this, when they are exposed to these theoretically new practices and protocols, their framework for knowledge doesn't set off alarm bells telling them that these practices are congruent with efforts to castrate, sterilize, institutionalize, or heterosexualize gay men and lesbians using intrusive, invasive, and unwelcome interventions.

They don't know as a matter of their training that the majority of gender questioning kids historically have grown up to be comfortable and well adjusted gay and lesbian adults. They have been trained, in fact, to see sex-role nonconformity or discomfort with one's natal sex as "gender" and to see this as a question separate from sexual orientation or identity.

Because of this widespread ignorance about medicalization in gay and lesbian history, well-meaning and otherwise competent medical professionals haven't connected the dots and said "let's slow this down."

Many well-meaning medical professionals also have interpreted "trans" as a natural extension of LGB issues. They wish to be part of the arc of history that bends toward justice. It has become very common for people to use the term "LGBTQ" in ways that suggest that lesbians and gay men are the same and that our interests are somehow the same as those of trans-identified people. While many of us have had histories of gender bending, gender play, and gender nonconformity, it is also true that gay and lesbian activists worked hard to end the medicalization of homosexuals; the current trans medicalization is the extreme opposite of this.

Very few medical professionals and therapists who consider themselves allies of gay and lesbian people understand this. They may even believe that trans identified males are lesbians, rather than heterosexually oriented men who prefer to look like women. They see medicalizing trans kids as somehow liberatory and an act of allyship with same-sex attracted people, rather than an alarming form of conversion therapy that is complicit with the destruction of gay and lesbian communities.

Many health care providers appear uncomfortable talking with kids and families about the possibility that the child is or will be lesbian or bisexual, and about how the family will nurture them should this be the case. When medicalization begins before kids have fully experienced puberty, or before teenagers have had romantic relationships, or are even comfortable discussing sexual issues, the question of sexuality can be cordoned off as something to be addressed later. By the time "later" comes, however, the young person's sexual functioning may have been damaged or destroyed, their fertility impaired, and their sense of self devastated by puberty blockers, cross sex hormones, and medically unnecessary surgeries.

What about the medical professionals and therapists who do have questions, the ones who are not comfortable prescribing experimental pharmaceutical regimens of incredibly powerful drugs to children, adolescents, or young adults with no verifiable need for them? If they are open about their questions, these professionals face ostracization from colleagues. They face transactivist efforts to destroy their reputations. They may be confronted as "transphobic." They reasonably fear job loss when working in environments that have become intimidated by trans activists or beholden to those upstream organizations that have pushed for the adoption of "affirmation only" practices.

Finally, institutional capture means you may be in a state in which laws have been enacted that position doing anything other than "affirming" immediately and constantly as "conversion therapy" — as though helping a girl become comfortable expressing herself in her body is bad medical or mental health practice. These laws mean that many mental health and medical providers fear not only for their jobs but also for their licenses. In such states, offering gender exploratory care or taking a developmental approach to supporting girls who say they feel like boys not only elevates the risk of a provider being treated as a transphobic pariah and made an example to colleagues, but also the risk that she or he will be reported to a licensing board for his or her views or practices.

Many physicians, psychiatrists, and therapists who are deeply skeptical about the "affirmation only" model have decided to keep their heads down and hope that, like the opioid crisis, this thing will eventually blow over and sanity will prevail. Unfortunately, damage continues to be done while they wait, and the fallout for the individuals and families affected, as well as for the broader society, will be long, painful, and expensive.

So, some of the providers in your world have adopted the assumptions of the trans affirmative model and have forgotten to treat your child holistically. They have forgotten what they know about both biological and psychological trajectories of human beings, and pass right over treating your child's anxiety, depression, autism-driven social challenges, and her trauma from bullying or sexual trauma or family discord. They don't explore whether your daughter is saying she's a boy or trans or non-binary to get a rise out of you, or to express the necessary adolescent rebellion from you. Others do have a critical perspective,

IT'S NOT TRANSPHOBIC TO SAY YOUR DAUGHTER IS A GIRL

but are uncomfortable saying so, and will refer you to someone else or wait for you to express some reluctance to buy in before they signal that they, too, have reservations. These medical providers and therapists, in many states, are living in fear of losing their livelihood.

This is what you need to understand, and this is why you need to empower yourself to take a very strong lead in protecting your child from medicalization. You will play a key role in freeing her thinking from sex destructive medicine framed as "gender affirmative care."

If you, like many parents, feel that your trust and your child's welfare have been betrayed by the health care system, schools, public policy, and the media in the throes of transgender ideology, you are not wrong and you aren't alone. You will need time and space to assimilate this information and a new perspective. Over time, you may wish to join others punching back against institutional capture. For some, this will be a necessary part of protecting your daughter in the short term. For others, it will be a political calling that you will take up later. For everyone, the first priority needs to be protecting the health, safety, and future of your child.

CHAPTER 5: BENT

Brave, Empathic, No-Nonsense, Trustworthy Strategies for Shielding Your Daughter

"I have heard their groans and sighs, and seen their tears, and I would give every drop of blood in my veins to free them."

— **Harriet Tubman, Underground Railroad Conductor**

Courage is the price that life exacts for granting peace.
— *Amelia Earhart*

Those who contemplate the beauty of the earth find reserves of strength that will endure as long as life lasts. There is something infinitely healing in the repeated refrains of nature—the assurance that dawn comes after night, and spring after winter.
— *Rachel Carson*

Ten years ago, if you had shared your worry about a daughter who liked to think of herself as a boy, resisted feminine clothing and preferred stereotypically male pastimes, I would have reassured you with the knowledge that most gender non-conforming girls experience a resolution of their questions about their sex, sexuality, and embodiment as they pass through puberty and the early adult years when human brains are still maturing. We would have explored whether your daughter was on the autism spectrum and feeling uncomfortable with peers, whether she'd had traumatic experiences that might make her feel unsafe being female in our deeply sexist culture, and whether she was anxious or depressed. I would have recommended treating any of these difficulties. I would have shared the expectation that treatment for social awkwardness, PTSD, or depression and anxiety, along with a healthy dose of reassurance from you that you were okay with your daughter turning out straight or gay, would help her feel happier and more at ease.

Otherwise, if your kid was already happy being who she was and her greatest issue was other people not being okay with her haircuts or clothing choices or rambunctiousness, I would have recommended we work on the homophobia and sexism around her, while trusting that she would grow into her own over the course of time without any particular treatment.

The behavioral interventions being used with gender non-conforming children in the US from about 1973 to 2018 were horrifyingly sexist and homophobic, humiliating and traumatic, unnecessary and ineffective; they were the behavioral version of today's sex-destructive medicalization practices. They didn't leave girls sterile, sexually mutilated, suffering osteoporosis, or living with male pattern baldness, but they were deeply invalidating and often inhumane.

For those reasons, I would not have recommended referral to one of the handful of pediatric gender clinics in the world: the Tavistock in the UK, the Karolinska Institute in Sweden, CAMH in Toronto, or the clinic in the Netherlands that had been rolling out the "Dutch Protocol." In hindsight, we would have both been glad not to have had your daughter seen in these places or others outside the US, as most now acknowledge that there is generally no long term benefit to medical transition for children.

Today, in 2023, what was true 25 years ago and 15 years ago and 10 years ago remains true: the majority of girls whose behavior doesn't conform to sex role stereotypes, even including girls who believe they are boys, will experience a resolution of their discomfort in adulthood. Many but not all of these will be lesbian or bisexual and will be grateful if they were allowed time to mature without invasive and irreversible medical interventions that would have caused myriad problems.

Unfortunately, in the last five years, the United States environment in which you, your daughter, and the professionals you trust to care for her has changed. Allowing puberty to proceed and work its millenia-tested albeit messy magic — the best strategy for most kids for a very long time — will now require heightened vigilance and sometimes extraordinary measures on your part to ensure that your gender-questioning daughter experiences a normal, non-medicalized course of development.

There will be widespread pressure on you and your daughter to subject her to medicalization, and immense social pressure on her if she is uncomfortable, bullied, has ADHD or OCD, has experienced sexual harassment or sexual assault, is on the autism spectrum, or is subjected to forms of misogyny that invalidate her as a girl in the context of the family. She will encounter other kids who identify as trans, see influencers enjoy attention for their medicalization, hear teachers, politicians, and activists collapse sex and gender and teach that some boys are girls and vice versa, and ask her about her preferred name and pronouns. She may have a girlfriend whose parents disapprove and who wants her to be a boy. She may conclude that life would be easier if she could become someone else, especially someone male.

She may be "socially transitioned" at school without your knowledge. Planned Parenthood may prescribe testosterone for her over the phone, without your knowledge. Depending on your state, you may lose permission to access her medical chart and therefore not know that a physician is describing her as a "transgender male" and referring her for interventions that will halt her puberty, masculinize her body, and set her up for increasingly invasive and harmful surgeries.

I review all of this bad news not to scare you, but to prepare you. If it appears that the way forward is through dense forest and difficult resistance, that's because it is: not because the core issues are impossible to remedy — which is not the case at all — but because of how the current environment makes those issues so hard to see and address.

Fortunately, you don't have to go it alone. Others have been here before you, creating a clearing.

Who Are The Girls Looking to Transition?

Before the rise of the new trans ideology, very few people sought transition. Most of them were adults and most of them were male.

Many of them, like Einer Wegenar, aka Lili Elbe, appear to have been men with a fetish known as autogynephilia. Some of them were gay men subjected to pressures to transition — this still goes on in some places in the world, such as Iran, where both same-sex attracted men and women face the choice of transitioning "to appear heterosexual" or facing a death sentence. Some were gay men who strongly felt life would be better living as women.

Very few adult women sought medical transition prior to the current moment, though many women have strategically passed as men for a whole host of reasons —often related to economies, jobs, educational opportunities, the desire to serve their countries, the desire to serve in resistance movements, or the desire to avoid male predation. Some women always have preferred a masculine aesthetic — unsurprising given longstanding differences in the functionality and quality of clothes designed for and marketed to men and women, and the thrill of subversiveness in a sex-ranked power hierarchy. All of this has been the case without medical transition. For lesbians in particular, as I pointed out in Chapter 2, much of the 20th century was spent asserting the right to be female and same-sex attracted without the torture of medical interventions.

20th Century girls who identified as tomboys — or even boys, unmodified —- often experienced no distress about being gender non-conforming. They were often brought to the attention of psychologists for their refusal to wear dresses or play with dolls by other people upset about their non-conformity. The standards for gender identity disorder of childhood, the backdoor strategy for treating kids who might grow up gay, allowed mental health workers to diagnose such girls and to "treat" them if a distressed parent or judgmental teacher made a referral. These treatments were designed to compel girls into "acting like girls" in conventional, conservative terms. This line of work clearly violated the APA's own standard of prohibiting the pathologizing of differences that represented a conflict between the individual and their society, but it appealed to conservative interests. Many such girls did eventually become distressed as a result of the horrifying and humiliating interventions to which they were subjected. Their distress was not a primary problem, as they were often comfortable with themselves — until medicine became involved – and they usually didn't seek transition.

In today's environment, we might think of two categories of girls who do seek transition.

One is the group of girls who would have been considered psychologically healthy but perhaps socially frustrated Tomboys of the late 20th century, girls who were comfortable in their skins and uncomfortable with the social limitations they faced because they were girls. Today, these girls are often described as gender distressed, rather than socially frustrated. In the context of big pharma, trans ideology, institutional capture and social contagion, they have been taught to interpret themselves as true boys in the weary old inversion model, recycled without evidence from the early sexologists. In the absence of alternative, material-based empirical narratives, these girls have been marketed an interpretation of their experience that tells them they are literally male, born in the wrong body, and in need of medical treatment. Unlike the 20th Century tomboy, the 21st century transboy has been marketed the belief that her body is the problem and sold the idea that the elective medical destruction of her secondary and primary sex characteristics will resolve her medically marketed discomfort she has been sold.

The second group of girls caught up in the medical momentum toward so-called transition is the group physician scientist Dr. Lisa Litman identified as girls experiencing Rapid Onset Gender Identity (ROGD) in a pathbreaking 2018 research article. These girls insist as adamantly as the first group that they are boys trapped in female bodies, but they demonstrated little evidence of cross-sex identification or even tendencies toward behaviors considered atypical for their sex prior to coming out as trans. Like the tomboys, however, these girls have been marketed both a problem and a solution that involves expensive medical interventions and the high risk of irreversible harm.

Girls in both groups have reported that they believed that they would be doomed to commit suicide if they didn't transition, and parents of both groups have been urged by ideologically captured clinicians and trans organizations not to question their daughter's claim that they were incorrectly sexed at birth, and to affirm their cross-sex identities with social transition and cross-sex pronouns.

Despite these similarities, among the two broad groups of girls caught up in trans ideology and the quest for medicalization, there are a range of paths onto the trail of trans. Here I will share some examples with the hope that they will clarify that your daughter's distress may lie deeper than her frustration over whether you will support her in transitioning. For example:

1. In the spring of 2023, a New York couple brought suit against their local school district for the intentional infliction of emotional distress in their 9 year old daughter. When their daughter'drew a girl saying "I want to kill myself," they discovered that the school had socially transitioned her without their knowledge, and had for some time referred to her as a boy named Leo. Investigating this, they discovered that a teacher had heard friends call the girl Leo— a reference to her astrological sign— and took this as a cue to start treating her as a boy. The child had demonstrated no confusion about her sex prior to six months of in-school social transition, but by the time the parents — who were reported to be open to sexual and gender diversity — discovered what was going on, their child reported feeling deeply confused about her sex and socially distressed. She transferred into a new classroom, where she was bullied by other children because the school had returned to using appropriate pronouns and her given name. The school administration acknowledged that it had long been aware that the original teacher frequently taught trans ideology outside of the formal curriculum and encouraged kids to experiment with "being gay" and "being the other gender."

In this scenario, we can observe the role of the social environment in creating gender distress. Only with careful exploration were the child's parents able to determine the root cause of their daughter's distress and begin to treat it — not with cross-sex medicalization but with trauma-informed care that affirmed and reassured her about *her sex*.

2. About a third of the girls referred for care at the Tavistock Gender Identity Disorder Service (GIDS) also met criteria

for autism spectrum disorder. Many detransitioners report meeting criteria for being on the autism spectrum, without having been diagnosed prior to transition. One of the high profile women who was medicalized in her teens — including with a double mastectomy — reports that she often felt uncomfortable in social environments as a child, had been distressed by the idea of puberty and sex, and couldn't imagine herself ever being as voluptuous as the celebrities she saw as embodying a beauty ideal for females. She reasoned that she might fit in better as a boy, and her parents were advised to affirm and to support medicalization, which they did. By 19, she was detransitioning, grieving the loss of her breasts, changes to her female reproductive and sexual organs, and the changes to her voice that resulted from the use of testosterone. She began to explore how her autism made her vulnerable to seeing transmedicalization as an answer to her questions about herself. In retrospect, the key developmental issues for this young woman were incorrectly coded as gender dysphoria and incorrectly treated with fast track medicalization.

3. Other detransitioners report that they were accelerated down the trail to transition *despite* deeply challenging histories with sexual abuse, sexual assault, disrupted attachment, obsessive compulsive disorder, dissociative disorders, personality disorders, family discord, depression, and anxiety that had gone untreated. The ideological response to these concerns seems to be that these issues will resolve after the person's body is changed with sex destructive interventions in the quest to become a different person, one of the opposite sex. Both trans identified adults who live as the opposite sex and detransitioners confirm that *transition does not resolve these mental health problems.* For many, transition interventions complicate and worsen mental health struggles as well as life struggles.

4. Homophobia is alive and well, and it plays a role in the decision of some same sex attracted girls and women to transition. In families with hypermasculine or misogynist men in the father's role, girls' gender non-conformity may not be tolerated, as appears to have been the case with the first adolescent girl transitioned under the Dutch Protocol, as

reported by sociologist Michael Biggs. Others report pressure from girlfriends or partners to transition. Lesbian transman Scott Newgent, an activist against child transition, reports that an adult female partner was deeply homophobic and her family deeply religious. Scott recounts buying a vision of how normal their lives would be if he transitioned, a decision he reports deeply regretting.

As alarming and confusing as it can be to hear your daughter insist that she is male and will experience terrible consequences if she doesn't have access to medicalization – or will impose terrible consequences on you — it is important to ask what the story beneath the story is. You'll need to understand not only the forces and influences pushing and pulling your daughter down the trans trail, but also her deeper vulnerabilities to gaslighting, manipulation, disinformation, and to adopting beliefs that are either wildly magical or overly literal, such as that transition makes a person the opposite sex.

In order to make it more possible to both stop the progression of harm and to sort out what else is happening. Here are 14 specific strategies parents have used to help girls redirect from the transition path:

1. Get her off of social media.
2. *Provide accurate, clear, precise, scientifically correct education about sex, sexuality, and sex-destructive medicine.*
3. *Deepen her connections with family members, pets, and other trustworthy adults.*
4. *Reconnect her with Nature.*
5. *Find the right therapists.*
6. *Help her reconnect with her own body.*
7. *Curate her school or educational experience, going as far as homeschooling, if necessary.*
8. *Curate her experiences with health care providers.*
9. *Supporting her development of critical thinking.*
10. *Teach her distress tolerance and resilience skills.*

11. *Help her feel empowered in her female body.*
12. *Support her in researching and arguing for and against possible options to problems, including her distress about her sex.*
13. *Reclaim sex-based and realistic language.*
14. *Infuse your daughter's world with images and stories of historical and contemporary women who are known for their courage, brilliance, strength and fortitude.*

In the next section of his chapter, I'll elaborate on each of these 14 strategies.

Breaking Up with Social Media.

There are five good reasons to get your child off of social media:

1. This is likely where she has been recruited or indoctrinated into the belief that she is trans and that trans medicine will solve her problems.
2. The activists in trans spaces online lovebomb kids and encourage distrust of parents, leading them to feel that the people who really love them are the trans community online.
3. Social media reinforces the gaslighting language of trans ideology, and your child doesn't yet have the critical analysis skills to sort ideological disinformation from verifiable information.
4. The online world is disembodied and reinforces your child's disconnection from Nature, friends, family, and her body.
5. When your daughter has doubts or questions about transitioning, and turns to online resources for answers, those "resources" will affirm her trans-ness rather than encourage her to explore her doubts.

Sex Education

You will need to undertake frank, age appropriate conversations with your child about the verifiable material realities of sex, sexual identity, sexual attraction and sexual boundaries. Make it safe and low key to have these conversations, so that you can ask questions together in an environment that is curious rather than judgmental. For example, when your daughter says "Sandy used to be a girl but is now a boy" and I think I might be too," responding with "that's interesting about Sandy. I'm sure you're a girl, but I wonder what you're feeling about what it means to be a boy. Maybe we can look at some drawings about sex differences to see how males and females differ."

With older kids, use more technical teaching tools, and remember to focus on sex, not gender. Use everyday life examples as teaching opportunities —- pets are neutered or spayed without being considered to have changed sex, plants in the garden and animals at the zoo all have sex differences and reproductive processes independent of how they identify. When someone talks about top surgery, correct them w/the medical term; the same with "bottom surgery. Seek out technical visual examples of these surgeries so that your daughter is exposed to more than the benign sounding terms that cover the medical realities.

When someone misuses the word "gender" when referring to sex, point this out to your daughter. Maybe even make a game of giving her a dollar every time she notices someone or something – such as a medical form — making this error.

Reconnect with Others

The isolation of toxic relationships shifts people's perceptions of reality and allows abusers — whether toxic partners or cult leaders — to control narratives in ways that serve them. When people spend time with others outside of the captured bubble, they begin to imagine other possibilities, test reality, and discover that they can feel less stressed in environments that don't require that they only reproduce or reinforce the ideological narrative. Helping your child reconnect to adults who have confirmed to you that they will not reinforce your child's misunderstandings about sex and gender if the subject comes up, but will relate with them around fun, learning, shared interests, holidays, and volunteer activities, can be very soothing and counterbalancing.

Reconnect Her with Nature

Getting your daughter outside, into Nature and involved with physical activity can also begin to re-ground her in her body, after years of pandemic-induced overuse of screens and the positive reinforcement she has received from pretending to be the other sex online. Camping is a great way to serve the purposes of getting into Nature with each other, and helping your daughter build confidence and joy in her body.

Find the Right Therapies

Given the prevalence of co-occurring conditions experienced by girls with gender dysphoria, it would be very helpful for your daughter to receive assessment and support from a competent therapist. Given the pressures on therapists to only affirm, and the ideological capture of many, selecting a therapist must be carefully done. If a therapist has finished training in the last five years, chances are that they graduated from an institution that was vulnerable to institutional capture. You must very carefully select any mental health provider your daughter sees. Gender Exploratory therapists use an approach that is neither affirmation only nor conversion therapy, and generalist therapists who have more than a decade in mainstream modalities are likely to be helpful —- their skills are often aligned with gender exploratory therapy. Practitioners of trauma-informed care, EMDR, and body-based interventions may also be good candidates. Certified Equine Gestalt Therapists offer the advantage of getting kids outside and connected to horses, and many have a special affinity for youth on the autism spectrum. Any therapist you choose needs to be carefully screened by you before you entrust your daughter's care to him or her, given how complex the professional and political climates have become around issues of gender. Pay for an hour with them before introducing your child, or decide to work with a therapist yourself for the purpose of getting coaching on how to help your daughter with her mental health issues.

Curate Her Education

In addition to reducing or eliminating social media from your daughter's life, assuring that she is not being socially transitioned at school may be your greatest challenge. Many districts or individual schools have adopted policies allowing kids to change their names and pronouns in school without notifying parents. Some have adopted policies punishing students who refer to others using sex-appropriate pronouns rather than chosen pronouns. Some districts have adopted policies that protect students from allegations of misconduct when they enter bathrooms or locker rooms of the opposite sex because of redefinitions of the words "male" and "female," and the displacement of medical, material standards by social identities — all often without parents' awareness or consent.

You will need to approach the school district administration, your daughter's school administrators, and her teachers to determine both policies around this and the content that's being taught. Once the situation becomes clear, you will need to make difficult decisions about how to monitor the school environment and your daughter's situation to protect her from ideologically-based education, such as the case of the 9 year old girl at the beginning of this chapter. Some parents transfer their daughters from public schools to religious schools, despite other philosophical differences. Some parents opt to home school. Others have decided to leave the country, looking for educational opportunities in foreign schools with conventional curricula and cultures. .

Connect with an Honest Doctor or NP

As with therapists, you will need to screen health care providers very carefully. Knowing the laws in your state regarding the misnamed "conversion therapy" and parental rights will be helpful to you, but you will still need to ask physicians whether there are policies in their practice that require them to affirm the cross-sex identity of a child, refer such a kid to a gender clinic, start the child on blockers or cross sex hormones, or register the child as a "transgender male" in the medical chart. You need to know if the health care worker will report you to CPS if you don't agree to sex-destructive care. Increasingly physicians are waking up to the reality that the practices that constitute so-called "gender affirming care" are not grounded in strong evidence of their benefit and are, indeed, experimental and illogical. When you indicate to a physician that you have reservations about medicalization, you will be able to assess whether they do too and are comfortable taking non-invasive approaches to your child's gender dysphoria or sexual uncertainty.

When your daughter has established care with a physician you trust, you may want to enlist that person in exploring your daughter's questions about whether she is male or female. For example, ask her pediatrician to run labs or conduct a physical exam to determine or confirm her sex and discuss the results with her. Always reorienting the conversation to sex reduces the wobble introduced by the indeterminate term "gender."

Make sure that your daughter is not recorded as a "transgender male" in the "SOGI" area of her medical chart, and that male pronouns are not indicated on her chart. Ask treaters directly at every visit "has anybody entered any SOGI data on my child's chart?" Also make sure you know at what age you will automatically be unable to access the parts of your daughter's chart that refer to sexual health. When that time comes, ask your daughter to sign a consent form allowing you full access to her chart.

Critical Thinking

Until humans achieve some semblance of biological maturity deep in their twenties, they are, somewhat ironically, prone to seeing the world in very black and white terms. This cognitive pattern inclines young people to code the world around them in terms of "boy things" and "girl things" and male traits" and "female traits." This tendency, and the immature critical thinking skills typical of childhood and adolescence, make young people vulnerable to manipulation by people who are more experienced, more cunning, and motivated by antisocial goals. While shielding your daughter from manipulation is crucial at the moment, supporting her development of critical thinking and more complex analytical skills will help her to build a cognitive immune system that makes her less vulnerable when she does encounter gaslighting, disinformation, and implausible claims.

Hans Christian Andersen's *Emperor's New Clothes* famously illustrates for children how easy it is for populations to fall into group think; accounts of medical scandals such as the US public health-backed Tuskegee Syphilis Study, the chemical castration of WWII hero Alan Turing and other gay men in the UK prior to 1967 under the guise of treatment, and the widespread use of DDT in the US help older kids learn about critical thinking related to violations of medical ethics.

The social psychology research of Stanley Milgram and Philiip Zimbardo focused on conformity and compliance, which grew out of questions raised by German complicity with the anti-semitism, homophobia, and eugenics of the Third Reich, helps older students learn about compliance and about the importance of asking questions and registering objections. Certainly, current news coverage offers rife opportunities to check facts and compare angles. There are many ways to help your daughter learn critical thinking skills, and their importance cannot be overestimated in the process of helping her become a competent consumer of medical and political information.

Improve Her "Distress Tolerance"

When therapists say "distress tolerance," we don't mean that your child should be expected to endure meaningless distress. We do mean, however, that she will benefit from building strategies that allow her to soothe and calm herself, to put distressing encounters in their proper perspective, and to recognize what poses a threat to her welfare and must be addressed. When transactivists express great distress over being misgendered, or claim that misgendering is an act of annihilation, they give evidence of having very low distress tolerance – of outsourcing their stability to the rest of us. We all experience emotionally painful events, including confusing and upsetting thoughts and difficult interactions. Helping your daughter learn to work through emotional distress by assuring her that she is resilient, creative, and strong and by teaching her strategies for staying calm in the face of adversity will also help her to feel more empowered and less vulnerable in her female body.

Reconnect Her with Her Female Body

The female body is remarkable in its strength, responsiveness, sexual power, procreative capacity, ability to sustain life in the young, all while supporting the kinds of brains that solve complex mathematical problems, write award winning novels, and imagine how to restore our damaged planet. Help your daughter reconnect with the power and grace of her body by providing opportunities for movement training — self defense and martial arts, tomboy pilates, weight training, hip hop dance, backpacking, cross country walking, horsemanship training, dog agility training, and swing dance that allows dancers to learn how to both lead and follow all help people be in their bodies. The more you do these with her, the more they will also help you connect.

Lead with Kindness, Curiosity, Creativity, and Science

Understand that your child is going through something difficult that needs to be treated with empathy and kindness. She believes she knows the solution to her problems. Harsh responses on your part likely entrench her position, encourage her to retreat toward people who "affirm" her ideologically driven conclusions, and position herself as victimized by you. You can firmly hold the position that you won't support further medicalization until she's older or until you both have a deeper understanding of the problems and solutions, while conveying curiosity and empathy. Engage her with statements such as "let's do some research on this."

Take her to libraries and teach her how to look for resources. Ask her to read medical reports and legal testimonies and discuss them with you. Reward her for writing "pro and con" papers in which she must argue for and against her own position on different elements of transition medicine. An example would be to ask her to write papers on how "Puberty Blockers are Helpful" and on how "Puberty Blockers are Harmful," based on evidence that has been verified. Teach her that when we buy a car, we do a lot of research. When we make healthcare decisions, we need to do even more. Offer her incentives to sit with you and watch documentaries that explore the challenges of medicalization, gender non-conformity across cultures, the state sanctioned transition of gay people in Iran.

Discuss what you learn and what she learns, as you continue to help her build critical thinking skills and a science-minded approach to evaluating all of her choices. . Remember that you can – and must —

listen to and validate her feelings, and can do this without endorsing her interpretations of situations or her ideas about the best course of action.

Use Accurate, Realistic, Sex-based, Non-ideological Language

As a gender scholar, it pains me to recommend eliminating the word "gender" from your vocabulary, but it is immensely clarifying in communication to do so. When you're talking about embodiment, always talk about sex. Return to the language of sex roles and sex role nonconformity, sex based rights, and single sex spaces. Challenge the misuse of "gender" for "sex" and ask your daughter to communicate her meanings without using the word "gender." Make sure to accurately name cross-sex hormones as cross sex hormones, rather than "hormone replacement therapy," to use accurate language for bodily functions such as breastfeeding, and to talk about transition and gender affirming care in ways that accurately reflect these practices. "Transition" isn't accurate because humans can change their appearance but not their actual sex. As we have said :gender affirming" is a lovely phrase but can't be empirically supported. These sex destructive interventions, rooted in homophobia and misogyny, are always elective procedures and never life-saving.

Introduce Her to the Legacy of Female Badassity.

Finally, you can help your daughter by providing her with diverse models of women badasses — those who engaged in acts of courage that changed the world and those that engage in acts of courage every day to care for and protect their families. Expose her to female rulers, female fighters, female peacemakers, female revolutionaries, female undercover crossdressing members of resistance movements, female scientists, female athletes, female postal carriers, female jockeys, female cowboys, female underground railroad conductors, female doctors, female lawyers, and lots of badass lesbians. Whether your daughter turns out to be a lesbian or not, knowing about the ways lesbian women specifically have contributed to making the world a better place for all women, against great odds, will help her envision a future in which she, too, is a brave and courageous woman, and will help her appreciate the everyday courage of all the women around her.

IT'S NOT TRANSPHOBIC TO SAY YOUR DAUGHTER IS A GIRL

There is no question that girls are deeply distressed. We need to work to understand girls' very real anxieties and despair. We need to give them the tools they need to understand the world and cultivate their power to make it a better place for themselves. Distressed girls need care and comfort and hope, models of female badassity, accurate information, and space to explore their hopes and fears. They need space to build skills at self soothing and distress tolerance. They need practice in setting boundaries and respecting others' boundaries. They need training in critical thinking, so that they know how to evaluate whether the emperor really is wearing new clothes, and they need training in resisting authoritarian propaganda. They need to read George Orwell and to discuss reproduction and anatomy in clinical terms.

Distressed girls need to explore possibilities for themselves without committing to courses of action which they cannot change. The strategies I named above — create these spaces and opportunities. The final strategy — exposing your daughter to the often hidden histories of strong, powerful, brilliant, courageous women who defied sex stereotypes and conventions — offers her visions of who she might become as a woman.

However you move forward, I hope you will give your daughter and yourself patience and grace. She has been directly caught up in this ideology through no fault of her own. Put the responsibility where it lies. You may also have been caught up, unaware of the pernicious belief system that has colonized LGBTQ activism. Be gentle with yourself too. Start where you are, honestly express regret or mistakes, correct what you can, and move forward.

I've started using the acronym BENT, in honor of our gay and lesbian resilience, to summarize an approach for getting girls to Adult Human Female.

We must be:
Brave and Bold
Empathic, Exacting, and Educational
No- Nonsense
Truthful and Trustworthy
BENT is a philosophical framework for responding to young people in distress, and also to ideologically captured professionals, family members, and friends. It's also not a bad life philosophy.

In the current environment it can require immense courage to say even obvious and simple truths.

Here are a few reminders of simple, obvious truths of which I can confidently reassure you. We humans are a sexually dimorphic species. Transwomen and transmen remain their natal sex. Sex is not "assigned at birth" but observed even before it, and is immutable. Cross-sex hormones and reproductive system surgeries don't cure emotional or social problems, and aren't medically indicated in healthy children and adults. "Trans" identity doesn't change one's sex, and can't be confirmed with medical tests.

"Gender" is not a biological feature of humans, so the phrase "gender affirmative care" is nonsensical and ideological — and its practice is sex-destructive. The same was true of so-called "cures and treatments" for homosexuality, which were the forerunners of today's sex-destructive interventions for gender non-conforming kids, many of whom are gay and lesbian. Trans medicine is deeply homophobic and sexist. Administering "trans medicine" to children and young adults as a cure for a non-existent medical problem or a mental health concern constitutes unethical experimentation. Children cannot give informed consent because they cannot yet grasp the impact of voluntary medicalization, including sterilization.

Adults are far better positioned to make competent decisions about their own bodies and the risks they wish to take on. When things look crazy, following the money will clarify the situation. Young people deserve better, and so do their parents. When the US has discontinued these practices, it is young people and their parents who will be left on their own to grapple with the fallout. Other countries with more rational and scientific approaches to caring for gender questioning kids are discontinuing medical interventions, having recognized these simple truths.

It is not transphobic to say your daughter is a girl.

Be BENT: Brave, Empathic, No Nonsense and Trustworthy. Holding ourselves accountable to this standard will help us all find a way forward.

RESOURCES

Thanks for reading *It's Not Transphobic to Say Your Daughter Is A GIrl: The Wise Lesbian Guide For Progressives*. To learn more about the topics I've covered and how to help your daughter and yourself, I've created a short list of resources that may be of benefit. You do not have to go it alone. To contact me directly, send a message to amberaltwrites@proton.me

Books & Articles

Biggs, M. 2019. Tavistock's Experimentation with Puberty Blockers: Scrutinizing the Evidence. Transgender Trend. https://www.transgendertrend.com/ tavistock-experimen -puberty-blockers

Biggs, M. 2022. The Dutch protocol for juvenile transsexuals: Origins and evidence. *Journal of Sex and Marital Therapy* 49(4):348-368. doi: 10.1080/0092623X.2022.2121238.

Biggs, M. 2022. Suicide by Clinic-Referred Transgender Adolescents in the United Kingdom. *Arch Sex Behav* 51, 685–690. https://doi.org/10.1007/s10508-022-02287-7

Barnes, Hannah. 2023. Time to Think: *The Inside Story of the Collapse of the Tavistock's Gender Service for Children*. Swift Press.

D'Angelo R, Syrulnik E, Ayad S, Marchiano L, Kenny DT, Clarke P. (2021). One Size Does Not Fit All: In Support of Psychotherapy for Gender Dysphoria. *Archives of Sex Behavior.*50 (1):7-16. doi: 10.1007/s10508-020-01844-2.

Dansky, Kara. 2021. *The Abolition of Sex: How the "Transgender" Agenda Harms Women and Girls.* Bombardier,

Davis, Lisa Sellin. 2021. Tomboy: The Surprising History and Future of Girls Who Dare to Be Different. Legacy Lit.

Dawson, Tracy. 2022. *Let Me Be Frank: A Book About Women Who Dressed Like Men to Do Shit They Weren't Supposed to Do.* Harper Design.

Dhejne, C., Liechtenstein, P., Bowman, M., Johansson, A. L. V. , Långström, N., Landén, M. (2011). Long-Term follow-up of transsexual persons undergoing sex reassignment surgery: Cohort study in Sweden." PLOS One 6(2): e16885.

Gans, Jared. (2023, May 6) Majority of Americans oppose gender-affirming care for minors, trans women participating in sports: poll. *The Hill.*

https://thehill.com/blogs/blog-briefing-room/3991685-majority-of-americans-oppose-gender-affirming-care-for-minors-trans-women-participating-in-sports-poll/

Hassan, Steven. 2015. *Combating Cult Mind ControlThe #1 Best-Selling Guide to Protection, Rescue, and Recovery from Destructive Cults.* Freedom of Mind Press.

Hisle-Gorman E, Schvey NA, Adirim TA, Rayne AK, Susi A, Roberts TA, Klein DA.2021. Mental healthcare utilization of transgender youth before and after affirming treatment. *J Sex Med.* 18(8):1444-1454. doi: 10.1016/j.jsxm.

Joyce, Helen. 2021. *Trans: When Ideology Meets Reality.* Oneworld Publications.

Knight, Kathryn. (2023, May 16). The stomach-drop moment I realised there was something terribly wrong at the Tavistock gender clinic: Nurse reveals why she blew the whistle on 'experimental' treatment on children as young as ten. *The Daily Mail.* https://www.dailymail.co.uk/news/article-12091229/The-moment-realised-terribly-wrong-Tavistock-Nurse-Sue-Evans-reveals.html

Littman, L. 2018. "Parent reports of adolescents and young adults perceived to show signs of a rapid onset of gender dysphoria." PLOS ONE 13(8): e0202330. https://doi.org/10.1371/journal.pone.0202330

Littman, L. (2021). Individuals treated for gender dysphoria with medical and/or surgical transition who subsequently detransitioned: A survey of 100 Detransitioners. Archives of Sexual Behavior.

Mills, C. Wright. (1959). The Sociological Imagination. Oxford University Press.

Orwell, George. Nineteen Eighty-Four. Penguin Classics, 2021.

Transgender Trend. (2019, July 1). The Surge of Referral Rates of Girls to the Tavistock Continues to Rise.

Kefler, Maria. 2021. Desist, Detrans, Detox: Getting Your Child Out of the Gender Cult. Independently Published.

O'Mally, Stella. 2023. What Your Teen Is Trying to Tell You: Surviving, Thriving and Re-connecting Through the Teenage Years. Swift Press.

Respaut, Robin and Terhune, Chad. (2022, October 6). Putting numbers on the rise in children seeking gender care. Reuters. https://www.reuters.com/investigates/special-report/usa-transyouth-data/

Reed, Jamie. 2023. I thought I was saving trans kids. Now I'm blowing the whistle. Los Angeles, The Free Press, 9 Feb 2023.

Sanger, Isidora.MD. 2022. Born in the Right Body: Gender Identity Ideology From a Medical and Feminist Perspective. Independently Published.

Transgender Trend. 2019. The Surge of Referral Rates of Girls to the Tavistock Continues to Rise. https://www.transgendertrend.com/surge-referral-rates-girls-tavistock-continues-rise/

Schrier, Abigail. 2020: Irreversible Damage: The Transgender Craze Seducing Our Daughters. Regnery Publishing.

SEGM. 2022. Fact-Checking the HHS: "Gender-Affirming Care and Young People" contains a number of errors and misrepresentations. https://segm.org/fact-checking-gender-affirming-care-and-young-people-HHS

SEGM. 2023. Transgender identity and suicide attempts and mortality in Denmark. *Elevated rates of suicide despite wide accessibility of gender transition interventions.* https://segm.org/transgender_suicide_mortailty_Denmark

Stock, Kathleen. 2022. *Material Girls: Why Reality Matters for Feminism.* London: Fleet.

Van der Kolk, Bessel. 2014. *The Body Keeps the Score: Brain, Mind, and Body In The Healing Of Trauma.* Viking.

Documentary film by self-proclaimed "West Coast Lefties:"

No Way Back: The Reality of Gender- Affirming Care. Affirmation Generation. 2023. Panacol Productions.

Organizations

Genspect: Advocating a healthy approach to sex and gender: www.Genspect.org

Gender Exploratory Therapy Association: A resource for gender exploratory therapists and families and individuals seeking them: www.Genderexplore.com

LGBT Courage Coalition: A coalition of LGBT adults concerned with pediatric gender medicine and the censorship of dissent. https://substack.com/profile/152060956-lgbt-courage-coalition

Our Duty: An organization focused on supporting parents and educating the public: https://ourduty.group/

Parents With Inconvenient Truth About Trans (PITT): Writing by Parents Struggling to Support Children Who Feel they are in the Wrong Body:https://pitt.substack.com

Rich, Adrienne. The Burning of Paper Instead of Children. Copyright © 2016 by the Adrienne Rich Literary Trust. Copyright © 1989 by Adrienne Rich, from *Collected Poems: 1950-2012.*

Sex Matters: An organization creating guidance and support for teachers, schools, media, academics, and activists because sex matters in law and society: www.SexMatters.org

Society for Evidence-Based Gender Medicine (SEGM). Aims to "promote safe, compassionate, ethical and evidence-informed healthcare for children, adolescents, and young adults with gender dysphoria." SEGM.org

The Lesbian Project: An organization working to improve and protect the wellbeing of same-sex attracted females, with the understanding that wellbeing involves more than equality: https://www.thelesbianproject.co.uk/

Transgender Trend: An organization advocating the safeguarding of children in policy and practice through the collaboration of parents, academics, and activists: https://www.transgendertrend.com/

Transition Justice: a legal non-profit connecting detransitioners with malpractice attorneys and helping them with legal expenses. www.transitionjustice.org,

Broader Activist Organizations Protecting Women's Interests:

Standing For Women: https://www.standingforwomen.com/ An effort to create spaces for everyday women to share what's happening to them --- which includes lots of concern about the medicalization of kids and public policy that affects women's rights to single-sex spaces, sports, services etc.

Women's Declaration International (WDI): USA Chapter: https://womensdeclarationusa.com/

Blogs:

Jennifer Bilik. The 11th Hour Blog. https://www.the11thhourblog.com/ Covers the intersections of transgender, technology, and capitalism, and provides a very macro and long-term perspective.

BROADview, by Lisa Sellin Davis. Providing "newsletter about the gender culture wars, & the history, science, psychology & politics of gender nonconformity—misunderstood by the Right and Left. Where do our ideas of normal for boys and girls come from? Speaking the unspeakable. Pro-complexity." https://lisaselindavis.substack.com/

Gendercriticalwoman.blog Examines "Gender Identity Ideology and its impact on Women's Sex based rights and Gay Rights. Explores how this has taken such a firm root in Western societies (Cognitive & Regulatory Capture)."

Kara Dansky's Substack. Dedicated to "Feminism and Fighting the Gender Industry." https://substack.com/@kdansky

The Stoic Mom Project. https://substack.com/@stoicmom.

Social Media Content Producers:

Benjamin Boyce: Interviews with professional researchers, psychologists, trans people and people who have desisted from transition. https://www.youtube.com/c/BenjaminABoyce

Exulansic: Exulansic studies trans ideology as a group of religious movements threatening our civil and disability rights and the medical consequences of invasive elective medical procedures under the umbrella of gender affirming care. https://substack.com/@exulansic

Utterly Moderate Podcast. The Utterly Moderate Podcast is "the official podcast of the Connors Forum for a Healthy Democracy. The core mission of the Connors Forum is to disseminate high-quality

Made in the USA
Las Vegas, NV
01 March 2025

18899902R00046